101
MUSCLE
BUILDING
Workouts & Nutrition
Plans

Acknowledgements

This publication is based on articles written by David Barr, CSCS, CISSN, Rob Fitzgerald, Matthew Kadey, MS, RD, Myatt Murphy, Jimmy Peña, MS, CSCS, Jim Stoppani, PhD, Mark Thorpe, Eric Velazquez and Joe Wuebben

Cover photography by Marc Royce

Photography and illustrations by Art Brewer, Michael Darter, Ian Logan, Erica Schultz, Ian Spanier, Larissa Underwood and Pavel Ythjall

Project editor is Joe Wuebben

Project creative director is KiWon Ballman

Project managing editor is Jared Evans

Project designer is Brandi Centeno

Project copy editor is Kim Thomson

Photo assistant is Erica Schultz

Founding chairman is Joe Weider. Chairman and CEO of American Media, Inc., is David Pecker

This book is available in quantity at special discounts for your group or organization. For further information, contact:

Triumph Books
542 S. Dearborn St., Ste. 750
Chicago, IL 60605
(312) 939-3330
fax (312) 663-3557
www.triumphbooks.com

ISBN: 978-1-60078-513-9

Printed in U.S.A.

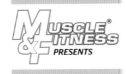

MUSCLE & FITNESS PRESENTS

101
MUSCLE
BUILDING
Workouts & Nutrition
Plans

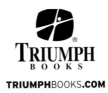

TRIUMPH
BOOKS

TRIUMPHBOOKS.COM

Contents

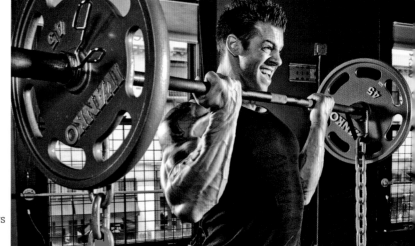

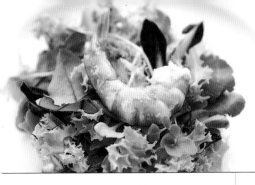

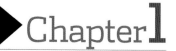

Chapter 1

Return of the King

Pay homage to the iconic barbell by remastering the moves in this old-school bash

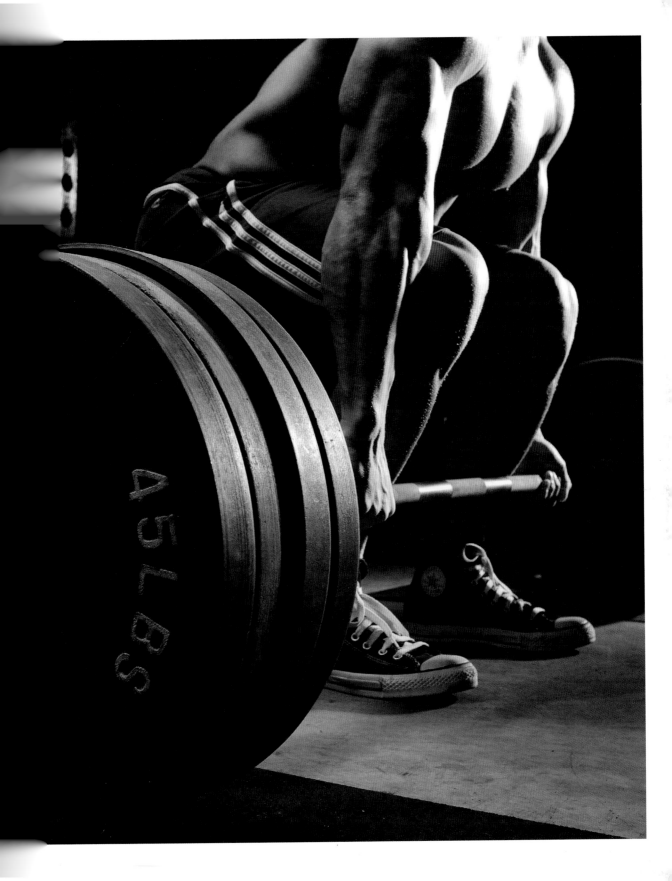

WHEN MAN INVENTED THE WHEEL — when he rounded off the square corners of some stone and realized it could easily be rolled from one place to another — he knew he was on to something. Since then, we've figured out how to cover wheels with rubber, combine them with internal combustion engines and move ourselves across land with an ease their original inventor would never have imagined. Yet the wheel's original design hasn't changed. It's still round, it still rolls, and physics continues to defy us to come up with anything better while still bound by the laws of gravity.

It's unclear exactly who first conceived the barbell, but there came a time when someone with some modicum of ingenuity (perhaps an Athenian who had a bone to pick with a Spartan who had kicked sand in his face) decided to slide weighted discs onto the ends of a rod and lift it in a variety of ways to get stronger.

"In the history of physical training, I don't think there has ever been anything that has improved upon the adjustable barbell," says Dan John, an author, national-level discus-thrower, coach and Olympic lifting advocate. "If it's too heavy, you take off weight. If it's too light, you add some. [Yet] people look at this like it's the Riddle of the Sphinx."

In the history of physical training, I don't think there has ever been anything that has improved upon the adjustable barbell

Maybe this decidedly old-school genius, whoever he was, had it right the first time. Maybe progress with the barbell should've stopped before things got out of hand. Since that initial barbell built its first set of biceps, we've seen an astounding procession of so-called upgrades. In trying to render obsolete the "hassle" of lifting weights with an actual barbell, these reinventions have convoluted our pursuit of physical advancement with all kinds of complicated contraptions, gimmicks and overpriced machinery.

Has any of this stuff really improved upon the original notion of picking up and putting down a barbell in different ways? To find out for yourself, locate a bar and some plates, and make that your gym for the next month. Put in an honest day's work with the one piece of gym equipment that has withstood the test of time and watch your training take off the old-school way.

"It's my belief that both athletes and fitness enthusiasts are capable of training at home at a level of excellence unmatched by most spas, gyms and training centers," John explains. "Contrary to popular belief, you can train very effectively with a minimal investment. I spent $159 on a 300-pound barbell set 20 years ago, and I can train for the rest of my life."

Add a dash of creativity to your training equation and there's little you can't accomplish with a bar and plates. In fact, when you designate the barbell as your main training tool, you'll realize that it's the machines that fall short compared to a simple barbell and a willingness to work.

PICTURE A LOADED BARBELL ON THE FLOOR. You can do three very basic things with it: You can push it, pull it, or combine pushing and pulling to accelerate it rapidly through space. In fact, every exercise you do in the gym can be reduced to fit into one of these three categories. The idea is to find the best combination of pushing, pulling and acceleration to gain strength, add mass, become a better athlete and increase your capacity to perform work.

"I assume only one piece of equipment with my program: a bar," John says. "Machines aren't the answer to your fat-loss or muscle-building questions. As a coach, I need to cut to the core of the things that work and repeat what works. Barbells work."

ROMANIAN DEADLIFT →

RDLs ARE GREAT FOR INCREASING HAMSTRING STRENGTH

Once you learn to manipulate the position of the bar with respect to your body — for example, figuring out how to squat without the luxury of a power rack or a set of squat stands — you can perform a seemingly endless number of pushing, pulling and dynamic-acceleration exercises with just a barbell and plates.

Presses, squats and extensions are examples of push movements. When you push a weight, in most cases you're fighting gravity by propelling a load away from your center. At the bottom of a lift, you're starting with your muscles and joints in a "coiled" position, and you're trying to finish the movement at full extension at the end of your range of motion. When you bench-press, for example, you extend your arms. When you squat, you stand up.

Rows, curls and shrugs are pulling movements, where you start at full extension, then close the gap by pulling the load toward a coiled position where the main joints supporting the weight are bent instead of extended. With bent-over rows, you initiate the movement with your arms extended, which is where the weight of the bar makes them want to stay, then pull the bar against gravity into a coiled position touching your midsection.

With Olympic lifts like the power clean and power snatch, proper technique combines both pulling and pushing to move a load quickly and effectively from point A to point B. These exercises work your entire body in myriad ways. Bearing a load and moving it repeatedly will make you stronger, but it's the nature of the movements — quick, compound and powerful — that recruits more muscle fibers. Along with the balance and stability these lifts require, that simply can't be replicated using machines.

In the program on page 13, each workout starts with compound, multijoint movements, then scales back to assistance exercises that help build strength and increase stability for your main lifts. Push and pull

**SPREAD-EAGLE
SIT-UP →**
Start: Load a bar with a 25-pound plate on each side and place it on the floor. Sit down and hook your feet under the bar, keeping your legs straight and spread as wide as possible. Lie back on the floor.
Execution: Crunch your torso up by bending at the waist and hips. Lower back down until your shoulder blades touch the floor.

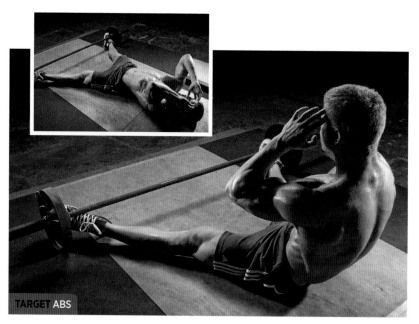

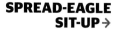
TARGET ABS

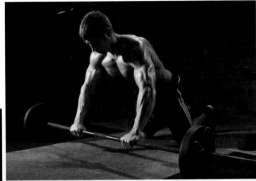

MIDSECTION MAYHEM
This challenging exercise will enhance core stabilization as well as hit the upper and lower abs

← ROLLOUT

Start: Place a barbell on the floor and kneel behind it with your knees hip-width apart and your toes on the floor. Lean forward to grasp the bar with a shoulder-width or narrower, overhand grip.
Execution: Keeping your arms straight, roll the barbell forward, using your abs to hold your body rigid, until your arms are fully extended. Contract your abs to reverse the motion.

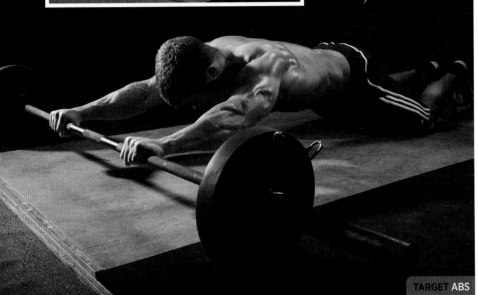

TARGET **ABS**

STANDING OVERHEAD TRICEPS EXTENSION →

Start: Perform a clean, then press the bar overhead using a grip just inside shoulder width.
Execution: Bend your elbows to lower the weight behind your head without moving your upper arms; make sure your elbows remain pointed forward or slightly to the sides. Return the bar to the start position by extending your arms overhead.

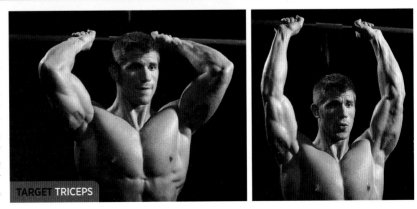

TARGET **TRICEPS**

moves are combined to target every main muscle group. On your lower-body days, you'll work the muscles crucial to deadlifts, front squats and Olympic lifts: abs, hamstrings, lower back and quads. On your upper-body days, you'll do a series of exercises for your pecs, triceps, lats, traps, delts and biceps. For challenging and comprehensive strength sessions, you won't need any more than this.

In the "Barbell Domination Routine" on page 13, the set and rep ranges we list are designed to cover all your bases: strength, hypertrophy, athleticism and increased work capacity. Understand, however, that these variables can easily be manipulated to meet your individual needs. To put on mass, add reps to each set until you're training in a range closer to failure. To get stronger, use more weight and fewer reps on your compound lifts at the beginning of each workout. To improve your conditioning, shorten the rest periods between sets.

Above all, embrace the barbell and everything it offers. It's humankind's original dedicated gym tool, and it's still the standard by which all workout equipment is judged — and found wanting.

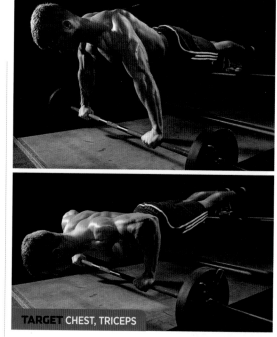

TARGET CHEST, TRICEPS

BARBELL DECLINE PUSH-UP ↑

Start: With your feet elevated on a bench, get in push-up position with your hands grasping a barbell at approximately shoulder width.
Execution: Keeping your body straight, bend your elbows to lower your chest to the bar, then push back up to the start.

"DEAD-STOP" LYING TRICEPS EXTENSION →

Start: Lie faceup on the floor with a loaded barbell behind your head. Grasp it with a shoulder-width or slightly narrower grip. Your elbows should point directly at the ceiling.
Execution: Extend your arms until they're locked out, the same as at the top of a bench-press rep. Bend your elbows to return the bar to the floor without bouncing.

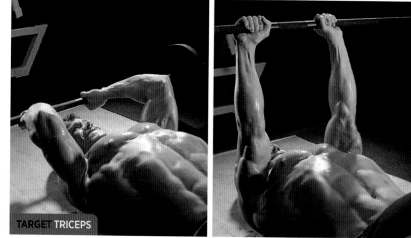

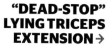

TARGET TRICEPS

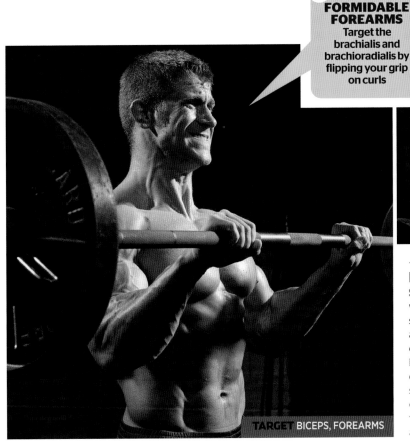

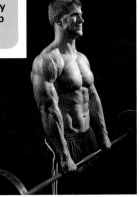

FORMIDABLE FOREARMS
Target the brachialis and brachioradialis by flipping your grip on curls

← BARBELL REVERSE CURL

Start: Grasp a barbell with an overhand, shoulder-width grip and let it hang in front of your thighs.
Execution: With your elbows close to your sides, bend them to curl the bar toward your shoulders. Return along the same path.

TARGET BICEPS, FOREARMS

BARBELL DOMINATION ROUTINE

MONDAY LOWER BODY

EXERCISE	SETS	REPS
Power Clean	3	5
Front Squat	3	10
Barbell Lunge	3	8
Snatch-Grip Deadlift	3	10
Rollout	3	15

TUESDAY UPPER BODY

EXERCISE	SETS	REPS
Barbell Decline Push-Up	3	20
Standing Overhead Triceps Extension	3	10
Bent-Over Row	3	10
Shrug	3	20
Barbell Curl	3	10

THURSDAY LOWER BODY

EXERCISE	SETS	REPS
Power Snatch	3	5
Deadlift	3	10
Good Morning	3	10
Romanian Deadlift	3	10
Spread-Eagle Sit-Up	3	20

FRIDAY UPPER BODY

EXERCISE	SETS	REPS
Military Press	3	8
"Dead-Stop" Lying Triceps Extension	3	10
Bent-Over Row	3	10
Upright Row	3	10
Barbell Reverse Curl	3	10

Chapter 2

Bursting at the Seams

If building muscle is your goal, this six-week strategy is all you need to achieve shirt-busting size

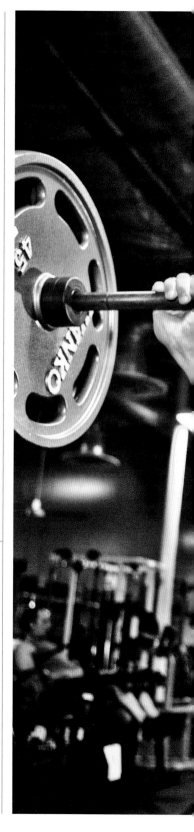

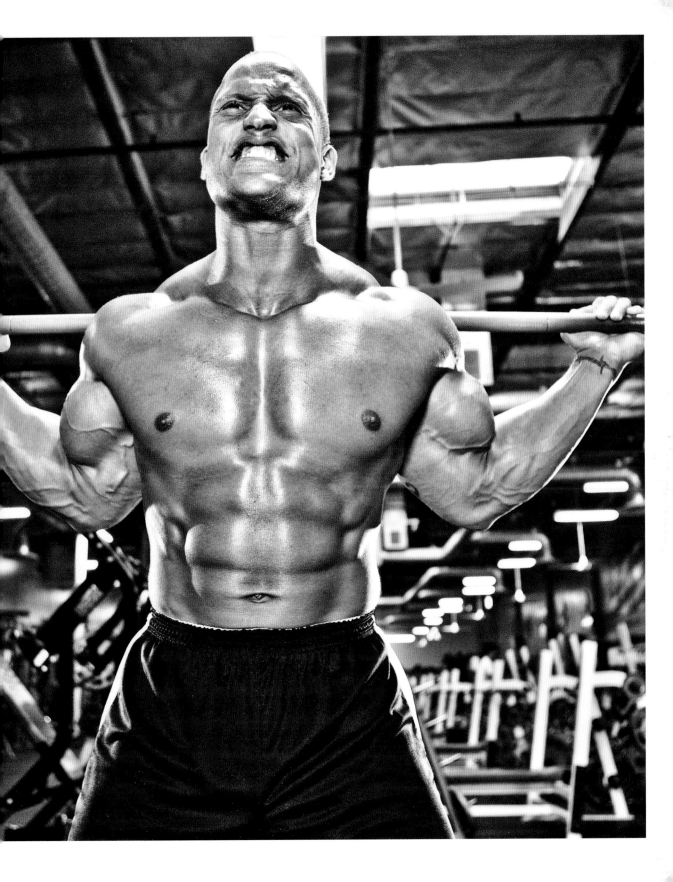

WHEN IT COMES TO PACKING ON MASS, the details don't matter so much. To gain serious size, you need to consider the big picture — the factors that have the most impact on shocking your muscles into new growth.

"Most guys assume the fastest route to bigger, stronger muscles is to work hard and lift heavy, but that's just one part of the equation," says C.J. Murphy, MFS, C-ISSN, co-owner of Total Performance Sports (total performancesports.com) and national powerlifting champion. Murphy's six-week routine consists of two three-week phases that incorporate a variety of exercises. "The best way to grow is to stimulate your big muscle groups, which triggers the greatest release of growth hormone," he states. "That's why each exercise is a difficult multijoint move that requires lots of muscle mass and tremendous torso stabilization."

That focus on your core is key. "Guys who want to pack on mass often do primarily multijoint moves for the upper or lower body, but they tend to neglect their cores because they assume training abs is unnecessary and will lead to a thick waist," Murphy says. "But if you're training to get big, all your

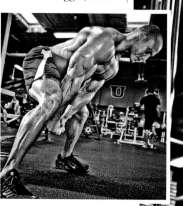

CABLE PULLTHROUGH
→

Attach a rope handle to a low-pulley cable and stand facing away from the weight stack, feet wider than shoulder-width apart. Keeping your back flat, bend your knees, lean forward and reach between your legs to grasp the rope with both hands using a neutral grip (as if to snap a football). Keep your arms extended. Plant your feet and stand erect, pulling the rope through your legs. Pause, then resist the weight as you return to the start position.

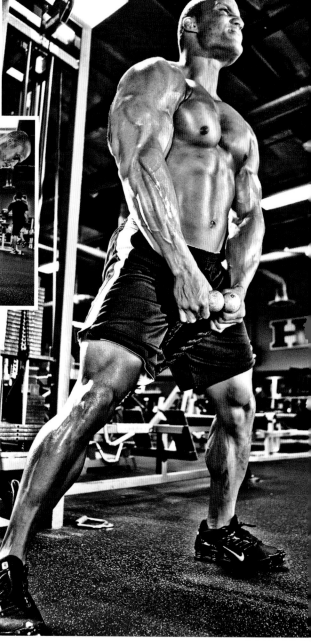

BACK EXTENSION/ROW →

Lie facedown on a back-extension bench and tuck your Achilles under the pads. Grasp a pair of dumbbells and bend over until your upper body is almost perpendicular to the floor; let your arms hang straight down. Slowly lift your torso until it's parallel to the floor, pause, then row the weights to your shoulders. Lower the dumbbells and return to the start position.

MASS-BUILDING WEIGHT PROGRAM WEEKS 1–3

EXERCISE	Week 1 SETS/REPS	Week 2 SETS/REPS	Week 3 SETS/REPS
DAY 1			
High-Bar Squat[1]	3/12	3/15 (add 10%)	4/20 (add 5%)
Dip (on parallel bars)	1/50	1/60	1/70
Weighted Back Extension[2]	4	4	3
Sit-Up	1/50	1/60	1/70
DAY 2			
Pull-Up	1/50	1/60	1/70
Heavy Dumbbell Walking Lunge	4	4	3
Dumbbell Incline Bench Press	4	4	3
One-Arm Barbell Deadlift	4	4	3
DAY 3			
Seated Barbell Overhead Press	3/12	3/15 (add 5%)	4/20 (add 5%)
Romanian Deadlift	4	4	3
Barbell Row	4	4	3
Dumbbell Step-Up	3	3	3
Windshield Wiper	1/50	1/60	1/70

[1] Place the bar high on your traps, with your feet shoulder-width apart. [2] Hold the weight behind your head.
NOTES: For exercises with one set, do as many reps as you can as quickly as possible, stopping just short of failure; continue until you complete the prescribed number of reps. Where you see four sets, do pyramid-style reps, increasing the weight after each set: 12–15, 10–12, 8–10, 6–8. Where you see three sets, do pyramid-style reps, increasing the weight after each set: 12–15, 10–12, 8–10.

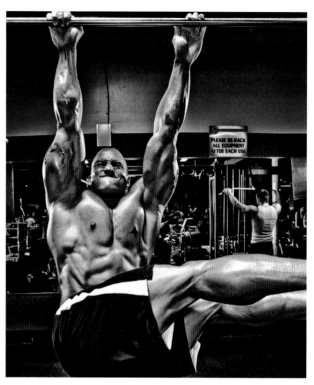

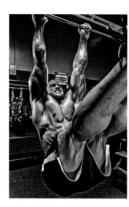

WINDSHIELD WIPER →
Hang freely from an overhead bar with your hands wider than shoulder-width apart. Tilt your pelvis upward and slowly lift your legs until they're nearly perpendicular to the floor. Keeping your legs together and elevated, rotate your hips to the left until your legs are almost parallel to the floor, then rotate back up and to the right. Once to each side is one rep.

MASS-BUILDING WEIGHT PROGRAM WEEKS 4–6

	Week 4	Week 5	Week 6
EXERCISE	**SETS/REPS**	**SETS/REPS**	**SETS/REPS**
DAY 1			
Low-Bar Squat[1]	4/6	4/8 (add 10%)	4/10 (add 10%)
Weighted Dip (on parallel bars)	1/50	1/60	1/70
Cable Pullthrough	4	4	3
Weighted Sit-Up	1/50	1/60	1/70
DAY 2			
Weighted Pull-Up	1/50	1/60	1/70
Heavy Dumbbell Reverse Lunge	4	4	3
Dumbbell Decline Bench Press	4	4	3
Dumbbell Side Bend	4	4	3
DAY 3			
Seated Barbell Overhead Press	4/8	4/10 (add 10%)	4/12 (add 5%)
Back Extension/Row	4	4	3
Barbell Shrug	4	4	3
Front Squat	4	4	3
Hanging Leg Raise	1/50	1/60	1/70

[1] Position the bar low on your traps and use a wide stance.
NOTES: For exercises with one set, do as many reps as you can as quickly as possible, stopping just short of failure; continue until you complete the prescribed number of reps. Where you see four sets, do pyramid-style reps, increasing the weight after each set: 12–15, 10–12, 8–10, 6–8. Where you see three sets, do pyramid-style reps, increasing the weight after each set: 12–15, 10–12, 8–10.

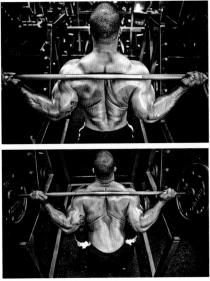

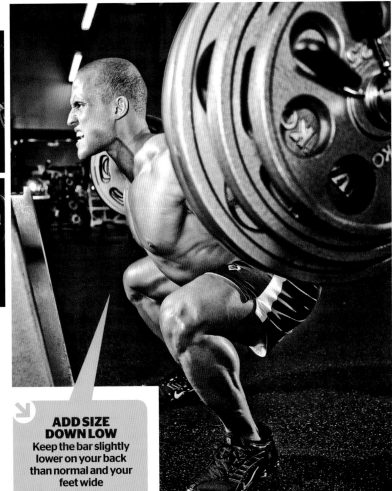

power gets transmitted through your torso." In other words, the stronger your core, the more effectively you can perform the exercises that will really bulk you up.

One thing you'll notice throughout the routine is a lack of isolation moves and supersets. "In a mass-gain plan, they'll only hinder your growth," Murphy explains. "Your agenda should be to work as much muscle mass as possible with as much weight as you can safely handle, and give your body enough sleep and food to grow."

ADD SIZE DOWN LOW
Keep the bar slightly lower on your back than normal and your feet wide

Rules of the Weights

RULE NO. 1: The main goal is to go as heavy as possible without sacrificing technique. "Choose a weight that makes the last two reps very difficult," Murphy says. "Each week you'll increase the weight by the percentage listed in the program [beginning on page 17]." If in Week 1 you squat 225 pounds for 12 reps, for example, then in Week 2 you'll add 10% (or 22.5 pounds). It's fine to round up or down so you're not trying to locate the 1.25-pound plates, he points out.

RULE NO. 2: If no reps are listed for an exercise, do them pyramid-style, increasing the weight after each set. You should get 12–15 reps on the first set, 10–12 reps on the second, 8–10 reps on the third and 6–8 on the fourth.

In Weeks 3 and 6, you'll do four sets of your first exercise, then drop to three sets for subsequent moves. "Since the primary exercises in Weeks 3 and 6 are the most difficult, reducing the number of sets helps prevent overtraining and injury, while keeping the intensity high," Murphy says.

RULE NO. 3: For exercises with high rep counts (50–70), work as quickly as possible. Start by repping to just short of failure, then rest. Continue until you complete the pre-

LOW-BAR SQUAT ↑
Place a barbell in a squat rack, grasp it with an overhand, wider than shoulder-width grip, then duck underneath it. Instead of resting the bar at the base of your neck, position it across the back of your shoulders and your middle traps. Step back from the rack and stand erect with your feet wider than shoulder-width apart. With a flat back, descend until your thighs are almost parallel to the floor, then push through your heels to return to standing.

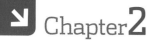

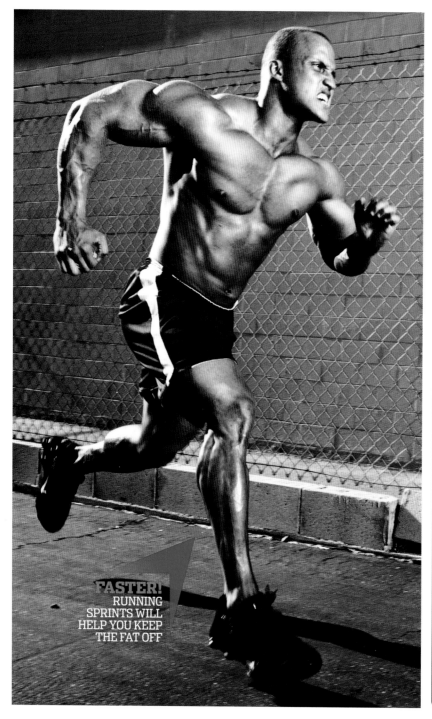

FASTER!
RUNNING
SPRINTS WILL
HELP YOU KEEP
THE FAT OFF

SPRINT CONDITIONING PROGRAM

The only "cardio" you should do during this mass-building program is a series of all-out sprints between weight-training days, 2–3 times a week depending on your fitness level. Here's how the plan breaks down:

WEEK 1	Sprint 20 yards x3 40 yards x3 60 yards x3
WEEK 2	Sprint 20 yards x2 40 yards x2 60 yards x2 80 yards x2
WEEK 3	Sprint 20 yards x3 40 yards x3 60 yards x3 80 yards x3
WEEK 4	Sprint 30 yards x2 50 yards x2 75 yards x2 100 yards x2
WEEK 5	Sprint 30 yards x3 50 yards x3 75 yards x3 100 yards x3
WEEK 6	Sprint 30 yards x2 50 yards x4 75 yards x4 100 yards x3

NOTE: Between sprints, rest no more than one minute to keep your heart rate elevated.

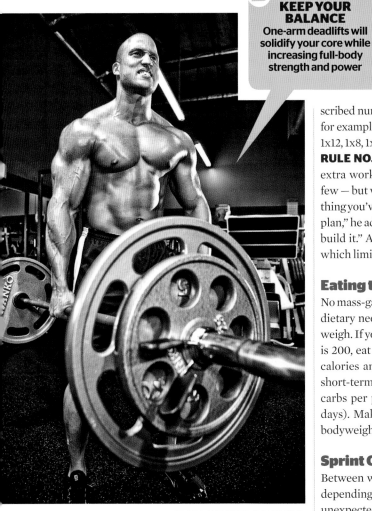

ONE-ARM BARBELL DEADLIFT ↑

Place a barbell on the floor and stand to the left of it with your feet shoulder-width apart. Keeping your head straight and back flat, bend your knees and lean forward to grasp the middle of the bar with your right hand. Your left arm should hang straight down. Stand up slowly, lifting the bar and keeping it close to your body, until your knees are just short of lockout. Pause at the top, then slowly return the bar to the floor. Repeat for reps, then switch arms.

scribed number of reps. If the workout calls for 50 dips, for example, your rep scheme might look like this: 1x18, 1x12, 1x8, 1x6, 1x3 and 1x3 for a total of 50 reps.

RULE NO. 4: "You must resist the temptation to do extra work," Murphy cautions. Stick with these very few — but very hard — moves, and hit them with everything you've got. "Don't do any traditional cardio on this plan," he adds. "You'll only burn muscle mass instead of build it." Also avoid activities that incinerate calories, which limits your growth potential.

Eating to Gain

No mass-gain plan is complete without discussing your dietary needs. In a nutshell, eat for what you want to weigh. If you currently weigh 170 pounds but your goal is 200, eat as though you weigh 180: Consume 20–24 calories and 1.5 grams of protein per pound of your short-term target bodyweight per day, and 3–4 grams of carbs per pound on training days (2.5 grams on rest days). Make adjustments to a new short-term target bodyweight as your bodyweight increases.

Sprint Conditioning

Between weight-training days — 2–3 times per week, depending on your fitness level — you'll do something unexpected: a series of all-out sprints to help condition your body to last through the six-week plan. "The entire program is intense," Murphy says. "So you don't want to do much cardio, but [it's still important that] your heart gets a workout."

Sprints also stimulate your metabolism, allowing your body to burn fat while adding muscle. "Although traditional cardio does little to boost your metabolism or build muscle, sprinting elevates your metabolism in the same way weight-training does," he explains. If you're worried about losing size, just ask yourself if you've ever seen an Olympic sprinter who wasn't jacked. Didn't think so.

The Mystery of the Pyramids

When it comes to building strength, few systems have proven more reliable than this age-old technique. A contemporary training twist transforms the well-worn classic into an invaluable asset

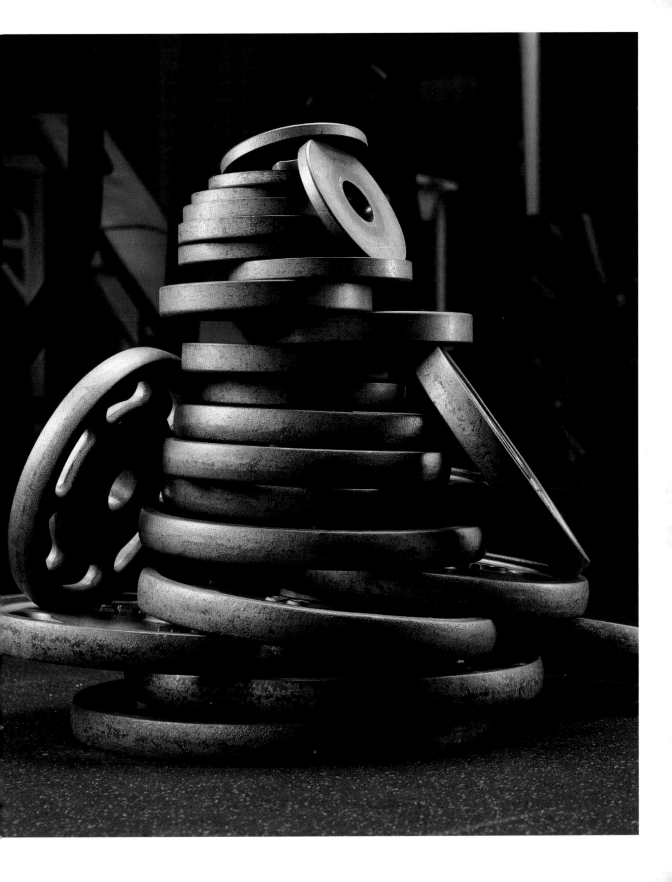

WE'LL TRY JUST ABOUT ANYTHING IN the gym to boost strength. From complicated fad routines to pseudoscientific lifting methodology, there's literally nothing that's out of bounds in man's quest to get stronger. But sometimes all you need to shatter a plateau is to go back to basics with a tried-and-true approach that possesses both scientific and anecdotal authority. Allow us to reintroduce you to the proven tenets of pyramid training.

When it comes to training for strength and size, few methods are more popular than pyramid training — for good reason. Whether you're a gym newbie, making a comeback to the weight room or an experienced lifter just looking to make some gains, pyramids deliver.

The genius of the pyramid technique lies in its simplicity: using progressively heavier weights on successive sets to prepare your muscles and joints for heavier work. But like many techniques, pyramid training has undergone some evolution over the years, incorporating tweaks here and there to fully exploit its muscle-building potential.

In addition to the bare-bones versions of pyramid training you're probably already familiar with — which we'll outline with beginner and intermediate programs in this chapter — we want to help you become familiar with the newest incarnation of pyramid training.

BASIC PYRAMIDING

The term "pyramid" refers to strategic and incremental increases and decreases in weight on a given exercise in each set. In its most basic form, a triangle pyramid, this type of training involves 3–4 sets in which you increase the weight and decrease the reps for each successive set. This slowly prepares the target muscles to use heavy weight; consider the early sets both a physiological and

neuromuscular warm-up that allows you to help avoid injury and move the weight with maximum intensity. Those interested in securing a solid pump or additional work can then add 1–2 back-off sets, in which you drop the weight and increase reps.

Another basic pyramid you'll find lifters using is the rack pyramid, a dumbbell-oriented skew on the triangle pyramid. You make the climb up the dumbbell rack, starting with light weight and moving up incrementally. The smallest increases are the most effective for volume purposes, and the goal is to work all the way up to a single, heavy rep, so choosing a good start weight is key.

TRIANGLE PYRAMID EXAMPLE

EXERCISE	SETS	REPS	REST
Dumbbell Curl	1	10	2 min.
	1	8	2 min.
	1	6	2 min.
	1	4	2 min.
	1	8	2 min.
	1	9	2 min.

RACK PYRAMID EXAMPLE

EXERCISE	SETS	WEIGHT (LBS.)	REPS	REST
Lateral Raise	2	15	10	2 min.
	1	15	10	2 min.
	1	20	8	2 min.
	1	25	6	2 min.
	1	30	4	2 min.
	1	35	2	2 min.
	1	40	1	2 min.
	1	35	2	2 min.
	1	30	4	2 min.
	1	25	6	2 min.
	1	20	8	2 min.
	1	15	8	2 min.

TRIANGLE WEEK

DAY 1: Arms, abs

EXERCISE	SETS	REPS
Biceps		
Barbell Curl	5	10,8,6,8,9
Dumbbell Incline Curl	5	10,8,6,8,9
Cable Preacher Curl	5	10,8,6,8,9
Triceps		
Pushdown	5	10,8,6,8,9
Smith Machine Close-Grip Bench Press	5	10,8,6,8,9
Incline Lying Triceps Extension	5	10,8,6,8,9
Abs		
Cable Crunch	3	8,10,15

DAY 2: Legs

EXERCISE	SETS	REPS
Leg Extension	5	10,8,6,8,9
Squat	5	10,8,6,8,9
Leg Press	5	10,8,6,8,9
Romanian Deadlift	5	10,8,6,8,9
Lying Leg Curl	5	10,8,6,8,9
Standing Calf Raise	5	10,8,6,8,9

DAY 4: Chest, shoulders, traps

EXERCISE	SETS	REPS
Chest		
Incline Bench Press	5	10,8,6,8,9
Smith Machine Bench Press	5	10,8,6,8,9
Decline Bench Press	5	10,8,6,8,9
Cable Crossover	5	10,8,6,8,9
Shoulders		
Dumbbell Overhead Press	5	10,8,6,8,9
Upright Row	5	10,8,6,8,9
Lateral Raise	5	10,8,6,8,9
Traps		
Barbell Shrug	5	10,8,6,8,9

DAY 5: Back

EXERCISE	SETS	REPS
Lat Pulldown	5	10,8,6,8,9
Bent-Over Row	5	10,8,6,8,9
Seated Cable Row	5	10,8,6,8,9
Straight-Arm Pulldown	5	10,8,6,8,9

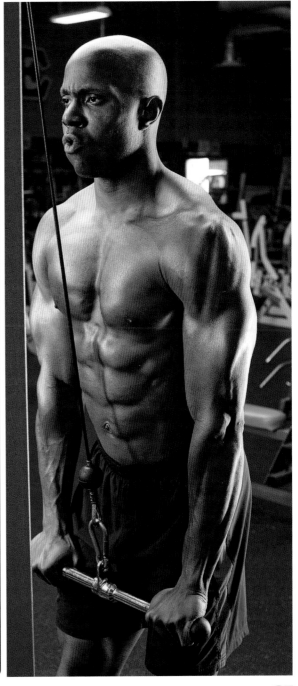

INTERMEDIATE PYRAMIDS

Building a solid foundation of strength with the basic pyramids will invariably leave you wanting more. The inverted pyramid and Oxford Method can provide it.

The inverted method is the opposite of the triangle: You start heavy, decrease the weight and then return to heavier poundages. The main payoff is that you tackle the heaviest weight right off the bat — after a specific warm-up, of course — when you're strongest. Your fast-twitch muscle fibers, which possess the most potential for growth, work overtime in the early sets, with the remainder of your muscle fibers coming more into play on each successive lighter set.

The inverted pyramid becomes more difficult, however, when you start climbing back up in weight. You should still aim to complete the target number of reps, which likely means you'll have to use less weight than you did on your way up. Because it's so difficult, most lifters don't use the inverted method.

The Oxford Method revolves around the same idea as the inverted pyramid: Go hard and heavy while your muscles are fresh. But unlike pyramids that are defined by ascending and/or descending reps, the Oxford Method employs one rep range for the entire exercise. This means you use the heaviest weight on the first working set before your muscles fatigue.

In the first set of this three-set pyramid, you use 100% of your 10-rep max (10RM), meaning you shouldn't be able to complete an 11th rep without assistance. On the second and third sets, reduce the weight just enough so you can complete another 10 reps. Keep rest periods

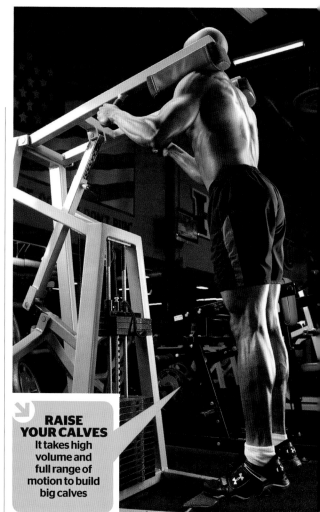

↘ RAISE YOUR CALVES
It takes high volume and full range of motion to build big calves

between sets to two minutes. At 10 reps, you're right in the middle of the hypertrophy range, only you're utilizing much more intensity. You can, of course, alter the rep range to suit your goals, using heavier weight and lower reps for power and strength, or higher reps and less weight for muscular endurance and calorie-burning.

INVERTED PYRAMID EXAMPLE

EXERCISE	SETS[1]	REPS
Smith Machine Bench Press	7	4,6,8,10,8,6,4

[1] Rest two minutes between sets.

OXFORD METHOD EXAMPLE

EXERCISE	SETS	REPS	REST
Pushdown	1	10 (100% 10RM)	2 min.
	2	10 (<100% 10RM)	2 min.

OXFORD WEEK

DAY 1: Arms, abs

EXERCISE	SETS	REPS
Biceps		
Power Rack Curl	1	10 (100% 10RM)
	2	10 (<100% 10RM)
Dumbbell Curl	1	10 (100% 10RM)
	2	10 (<100% 10RM)
Standing One-Arm Preacher Curl	1	10 (100% 10RM)
	2	10 (<100% 10RM)
Triceps		
Weighted Dip	1	10 (100% 10RM)
	2	10 (<100% 10RM)
Seated DB Overhead Triceps Extension	1	10 (100% 10RM)
	2	10 (<100% 10RM)
Reverse-Grip Bench Press	1	10 (100% 10RM)
	2	10 (<100% 10RM)
Abs		
Standing Cable Crunch	3	8,10,15

DAY 2: Legs

EXERCISE	SETS	REPS
Smith Machine Squat	1	10 (100% 10RM)
	2	10 (<100% 10RM)
Leg Press	1	10 (100% 10RM)
	2	10 (<100% 10RM)
Leg Extension	1	10 (100% 10RM)
	2	10 (<100% 10RM)
Smith Machine Lunge	1	10 (100% 10RM)
	2	10 (<100% 10RM)
Seated Leg Curl	1	10 (100% 10RM)
	2	10 (<100% 10RM)
Jump Squat	1	to failure
Seated Calf Raise	3	25

DAY 4: Chest, shoulders, traps

EXERCISE	SETS	REPS
Chest		
Dumbbell Incline Flye	1	10 (100% 10RM)
	2	10 (<100% 10RM)
Dumbbell Incline Press	1	10 (100% 10RM)
	2	10 (<100% 10RM)
Flat-Bench Cable Flye	1	10 (100% 10RM)
	2	10 (<100% 10RM)
Dumbbell Bench Press	1	10 (100% 10RM)
	2	10 (<100% 10RM)
Dumbbell Incline Pullover	1	10 (100% 10RM)
	2	10 (<100% 10RM)
Shoulders		
Arnold Press	1	10 (100% 10RM)
	2	10 (<100% 10RM)
Dumbbell Upright Row	1	10 (100% 10RM)
	2	10 (<100% 10RM)
Bent-Over Lateral Raise	1	10 (100% 10RM)
	2	10 (<100% 10RM)
Traps		
Dumbbell Shrug	1	10 (100% 10RM)
	2	10 (<100% 10RM)

DAY 5: Back

EXERCISE	SETS	REPS
Bent-Over Row	1	10 (100% 10RM)
	2	10 (<100% 10RM)
T-Bar Row	1	10 (100% 10RM)
	2	10 (<100% 10RM)
Standing Cable Row	1	10 (100% 10RM)
	2	10 (<100% 10RM)
Barbell Decline Pullover	1	10 (100% 10RM)
	2	10 (<100% 10RM)

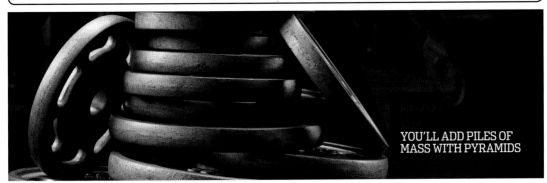

YOU'LL ADD PILES OF MASS WITH PYRAMIDS

ADVANCED PYRAMID

The inverted pyramid and Oxford Method are pretty tough in their own right, especially if you're unfamiliar with pyramids. But this program takes pyramiding to a whole new level.

Ascending rest-pause pyramids are a hybrid of pyramid sets and rest-pause training, which takes advantage of your body's immediate energy stores by training with heavier weight (but not to failure) with short rest periods interspersed throughout. This allows your body to partially recover its explosive energy stores for your next heavy set. The result is more reps with better form than you could handle in straight-sets fashion.

In your first set, select a weight you can manage for 10 reps, but do only five to stop short of failure and allow for maximum power recuperation. Rest for five seconds, then do five more reps. Rest another five seconds, then knock out a final five reps at that weight. That's one set.

Add 5–10 pounds on your next set (9RM) and move up the pyramid, completing four reps before taking a 7–10-second rest. Follow this pattern for your next two progressively heavier weight loads, with your rest periods stretching to 20 seconds. On your heaviest sets, continue performing sets of two until you can't do two full reps.

ASCENDING REST-PAUSE EXAMPLE

EXERCISE	LOAD	SETS[1]	REPS/REST (SEC.)
Seated Cable Row	10RM	1	5/5, 5/5, 5
	9RM	1	4/7–10, 4/7–10, 4
	8RM	1	3/10–12, 3/10–12, 3
	7RM	1	2/20 to failure

[1] Rest 2–3 minutes between sets.

STANDING BARBELL CURL
Keep your elbows in at your sides while curling to place all tension on your biceps

ASCENDING REST-PAUSE WEEK

DAY 1: Arms, abs

EXERCISE	LOAD	SETS	REPS/REST (SEC.)
Biceps			
Seated Barbell Curl	10RM	1	5/5, 5/5, 5
	9RM	1	4/7–10, 4/7–10, 4
	8RM	1	3/10–12, 3/10–12, 3
	7RM	1	2/20 to failure
Lying Cable Curl	10RM	1	5/5, 5/5, 5
	9RM	1	4/7–10, 4/7–10, 4
	8RM	1	3/10–12, 3/10–12, 3
	7RM	1	2/20 to failure
Smith Machine Drag Curl	10RM	1	5/5, 5/5, 5
	9RM	1	4/7–10, 4/7–10, 4
	8RM	1	3/10–12, 3/10–12, 3
	7RM	1	2/20 to failure
Triceps			
Pushdown	10RM	1	5/5, 5/5, 5
	9RM	1	4/7–10, 4/7–10, 4
	8RM	1	3/10–12, 3/10–12, 3
	7RM	1	2/20 to failure
Cable Overhead Triceps Extension	10RM	1	5/5, 5/5, 5
	9RM	1	4/7–10, 4/7–10, 4
	8RM	1	3/10–12, 3/10–12, 3
	7RM	1	2/20 to failure
Cable Kickback	10RM	1	5/5, 5/5, 5
	9RM	1	4/7–10, 4/7–10, 4
	8RM	1	3/10–12, 3/10–12, 3
	7RM	1	2/20 to failure
Abs			
Double Crunch		3	to failure

DAY 2: Legs

EXERCISE	LOAD	SETS	REPS/REST (SEC.)
Front Squat	10RM	1	5/5, 5/5, 5
	9RM	1	4/7–10, 4/7–10, 4
	8RM	1	3/10–12, 3/10–12, 3
	7RM	1	2/20 to failure
Hack Squat	10RM	1	5/5, 5/5, 5
	9RM	1	4/7–10, 4/7–10, 4
	8RM	1	3/10–12, 3/10–12, 3
	7RM	1	2/20 to failure
Leg Extension	10RM	1	5/5, 5/5, 5
	9RM	1	4/7–10, 4/7–10, 4
	8RM	1	3/10–12, 3/10–12, 3
	7RM	1	2/20 to failure
Romanian Deadlift	10RM	1	5/5, 5/5, 5
	9RM	1	4/7–10, 4/7–10, 4
	8RM	1	3/10–12, 3/10–12, 3
	7RM	1	2/20 to failure
Dumbbell Calf Raise		3	30

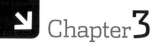
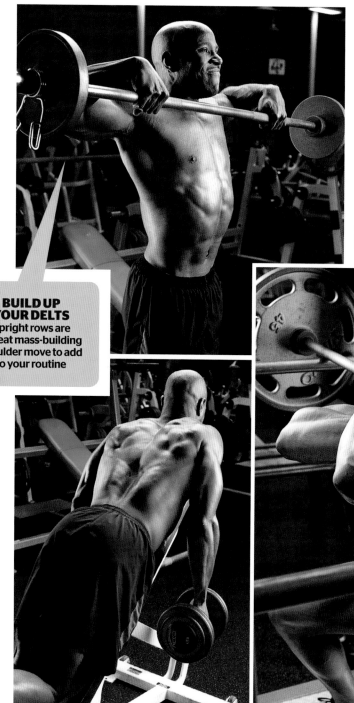

TRAINING SPLIT

DAY	BODYPARTS TRAINED
1	Arms, abs
2	Legs
3	Rest
4	Chest, shoulders, traps
5	Back
6–7	Rest

BUILD UP YOUR DELTS
Upright rows are a great mass-building shoulder move to add to your routine

DAY 4: Chest, shoulders, traps

EXERCISE	LOAD	SETS	REPS/REST (SEC.)
Chest			
Power-Rack Bench Press	10RM	1	5/5, 5/5, 5
	9RM	1	4/7–10, 4/7–10, 4
	8RM	1	3/10–12, 3/10–12, 3
	7RM	1	2/20 to failure
Dumbbell Pullover	10RM	1	5/5, 5/5, 5
	9RM	1	4/7–10, 4/7–10, 4
	8RM	1	3/10–12, 3/10–12, 3
	7RM	1	2/20 to failure
Weighted Dip	10RM	1	5/5, 5/5, 5
	9RM	1	4/7–10, 4/7–10, 4
	8RM	1	3/10–12, 3/10–12, 3
	7RM	1	2/20 to failure
Shoulders			
Machine Lateral Raise	10RM	1	5/5, 5/5, 5
	9RM	1	4/7–10, 4/7–10, 4
	8RM	1	3/10–12, 3/10–12, 3
	7RM	1	2/20 to failure
Seated Barbell Overhead Press	10RM	1	5/5, 5/5, 5
	9RM	1	4/7–10, 4/7–10, 4
	8RM	1	3/10–12, 3/10–12, 3
	7RM	1	2/20 to failure
Smith Machine Upright Row	10RM	1	5/5, 5/5, 5
	9RM	1	4/7–10, 4/7–10, 4
	8RM	1	3/10–12, 3/10–12, 3
	7RM	1	2/20 to failure
Traps			
Dumbbell Incline Shrug	10RM	1	5/5, 5/5, 5
	9RM	1	4/7–10, 4/7–10, 4
	8RM	1	3/10–12, 3/10–12, 3
	7RM	1	2/20 to failure

DAY 5: Back

EXERCISE	LOAD	SETS	REPS/REST (SEC.)
Rack Pull	10RM	1	5/5, 5/5, 5
	9RM	1	4/7–10, 4/7–10, 4
	8RM	1	3/10–12, 3/10–12, 3
	7RM	1	2/20 to failure
Wide-Grip Seated Cable Row	10RM	1	5/5, 5/5, 5
	9RM	1	4/7–10, 4/7–10, 4
	8RM	1	3/10–12, 3/10–12, 3
	7RM	1	2/20 to failure
One-Arm Dumbbell Row	10RM	1	5/5, 5/5, 5
	9RM	1	4/7–10, 4/7–10, 4
	8RM	1	3/10–12, 3/10–12, 3
	7RM	1	2/20 to failure
Pull-Up		1	to failure

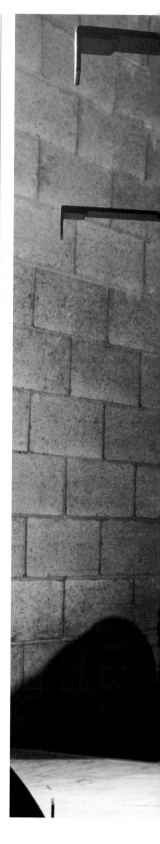

Chapter 4

Highs & Lows

Are you prepared to swap pain for results? If you have the intestinal fortitude to run through this variable rep-scheme gauntlet, your courage will be rewarded

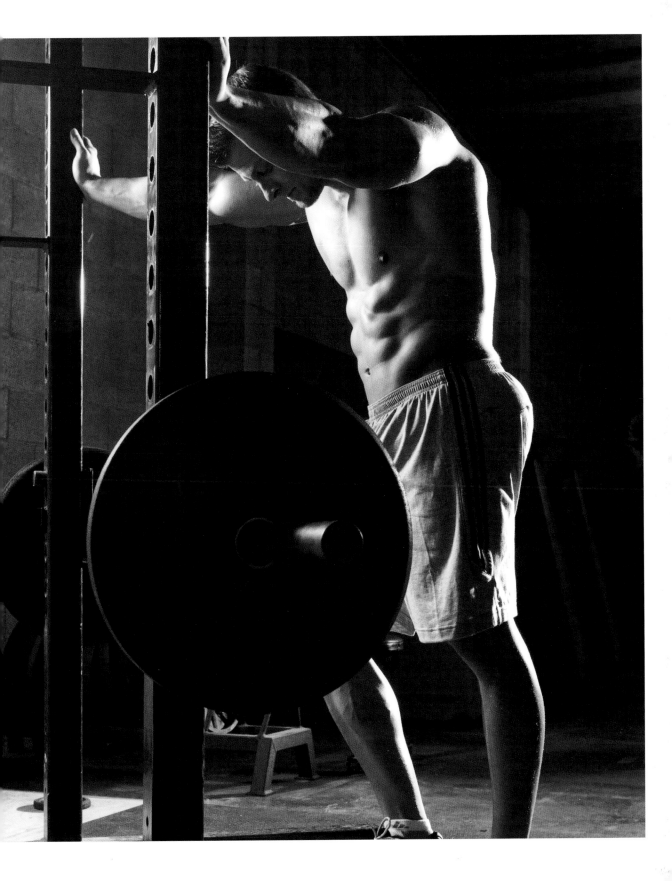

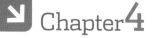

TWELVE OR MORE REPS FOR MUSCU- lar endurance. Six to 11 reps for size. Five or fewer for strength. These are the standard goal-based rep-range recommendations, and for most guys in the weight room, they pay dividends. But intermediate and advanced-level lifters can and should defy conventional wisdom from time to time in the interest of sustaining progress. By combining high and low reps in the same workout, you can reap the benefits that each has to offer while simultaneously boosting your metabolism.

But there's a catch: This is no cruise-control workout; it's unapologetically intense and far more demanding than many prescribed routines. While your time in the gym might usually be an escape from life's tensions, this "Highs & Lows" workout is guaranteed to put you under stress, just a different kind.

BEST OF BOTH WORLDS

Our "Highs & Lows" program is a widow-maker intensity-wise, despite its non-traditional rep scheme. Some people prefer to eschew high-reprange work altogether, figuring light weight leads to small muscles, or high-rep sets are just for burning calories. That's simply not true. High reps not only provide a fantastic pump but can also assist your growth.

While you'll perform sets of up to 24 reps in this program, you'll also blast through big-weight sets of 4–6 reps and moderate-load sets of 8–12. The intense pace of the workouts — there's little rest between sets — amps up your metabolism, all but eliminating the need for additional calorie-burning cardio.

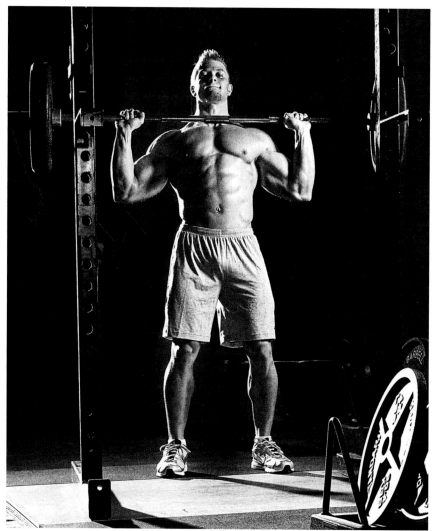

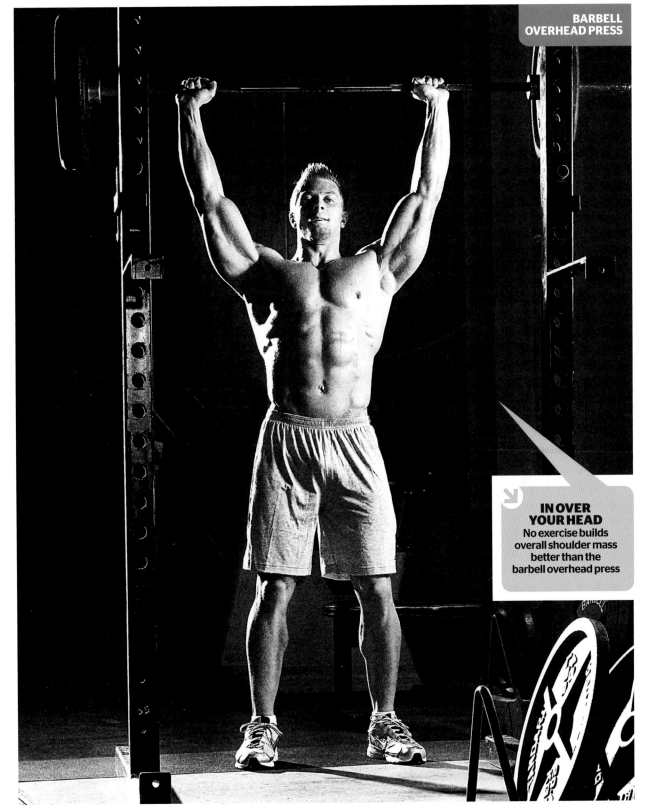

IN OVER YOUR HEAD
No exercise builds overall shoulder mass better than the barbell overhead press

In this program you'll hit each bodypart twice a week, which translates to six days in the gym. The good news is you'll start with only 1–2 working sets for each bodypart. The bad news is if you're used to doing 8–10 reps, each set will feel like a marathon.

In each workout you'll train for either strength and size (Days 1–3) or strength and endurance (Days 4–6). When training for strength and size, you'll top out at 12 reps and go as low as four. For strength and endurance, you'll go as high as 24 reps and as low as eight. Every set has two parts, each a mirror image of the other. The reps you perform in the second half of a set will be the reverse of the first half.

On a strength and endurance day, for example, you'll choose one pair of dumbbells with which you fail at 12 reps and one lighter pair for the high-end spectrum (24 reps), switching between the two throughout the set. In other words, you do your heavier set of 12 reps then dive right into your set of 24 reps with the lighter weights. Then you'll immediately grab your heavier dumbbells again and aim for 10 reps. Switch back to the lighter set and try for 20. Return to heavy for eight reps, then go back to the lighter weights with a target of 16.

Rest 2–3 minutes, then reverse the climb using the same weights. On the way up you did 12–24, 10–20 and 8–16, so on the way down you'll do 24–12, 20–10 and 16–8. That's one set. During a strength and size workout, you'll perform half as many reps: 6–12, 5–10 and 4–8 on the way up and 12–6, 10–5 and 8–4 going down.

Dumbbells are ideal because of the resistance and overall muscle recruitment they provide. Plus, you can grab two pairs of weights without being an equipment hog. Machines also work well because you can easily move the pin between rep ranges. We don't recommend using barbells because claiming two of them is a difficult score in any gym. But if you can get away with it, then by all means use them.

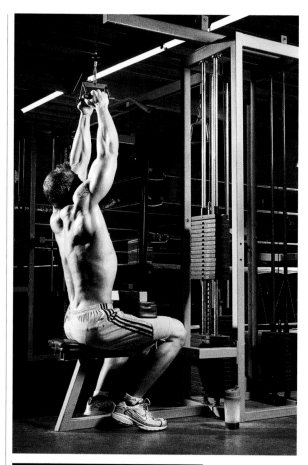

TRAINING SPLIT

DAY	BODYPARTS TRAINED
1	Chest, arms
2	Legs, abs
3	Back, shoulders, traps
4	Chest, arms
5	Legs, abs
6	Back, shoulders, traps
7	Rest

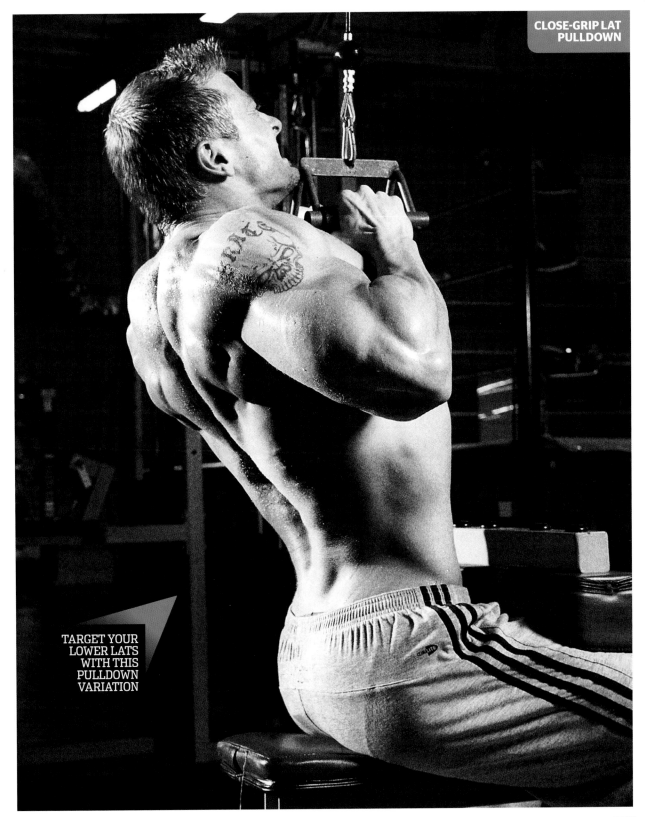

TARGET YOUR LOWER LATS WITH THIS PULLDOWN VARIATION

The program is progressive in that you add one exercise per bodypart in Weeks 3 and 4, nearly doubling the already substantial volume and pushing your pain threshold — and your metabolic rate — to the limit. By the end, you'll be doing 2–3 working sets per major muscle group per workout.

Utilizing both ends of the rep-range spectrum will help you build strong, dense muscles while whittling away bodyfat. Pair this with the nutrition and supplement advice in Chapters 14 and 15, and you'll enjoy a better body long after the pain subsides.

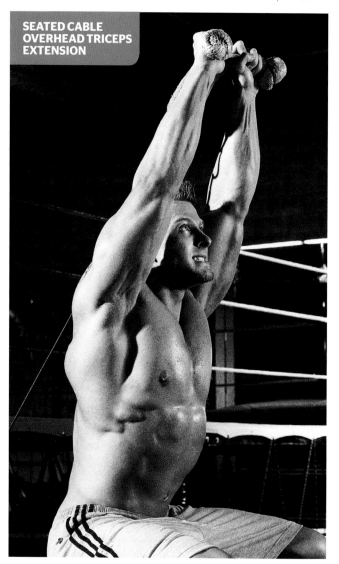

SEATED CABLE OVERHEAD TRICEPS EXTENSION

HIGHS & LOWS PROGRAM

During the next four weeks you'll hit each bodypart twice per week: One workout will be dedicated to strength and size, another to strength and endurance. Do a few warm-up sets for each bodypart, then dive right in to the Highs & Lows. The rep schemes are as follows:

→ STRENGTH & SIZE (S&S)

6 reps & 12 reps
5 reps & 10 reps
4 reps & 8 reps
Rest 2–3 minutes, then reverse
12 reps & 6 reps
10 reps & 5 reps
8 reps & 4 reps

→ STRENGTH & ENDURANCE (S&E)

12 reps & 24 reps
10 reps & 20 reps
8 reps & 16 reps
Rest 2–3 minutes, then reverse
24 reps & 12 reps
20 reps & 10 reps
16 reps & 8 reps

HIGHS & LOWS PROGRAM WEEKS 1+2

Strength & Size

DAY 1 Chest, arms

EXERCISE	SETS	REPS
Chest		
Incline Flye	2–3[1]	8–12
Dumbbell Incline Press	1	S&S
Machine Press	1	S&S
Biceps		
Preacher Curl	2–3[1]	8–12
Barbell Curl	1	S&S
Triceps		
Pushdown	2–3[1]	8–12
Cable Overhead Extension	1	S&S

[1] warm-up

DAY 2 Legs, abs

EXERCISE	SETS	REPS
Quads/Hams		
Leg Extension	2–3[1]	8–12
Leg Curl	2–3[1]	8–12
Leg Extension	1	S&S
Leg Curl	1	S&S
Calves		
Standing Calf Raise	1	S&S
Abs		
Machine Crunch	1	S&S

[1] warm-up

DAY 3 Back, shoulders, traps

EXERCISE	SETS	REPS
Back		
Lat Pulldown	2–3[1]	8–12
Seated Cable Row	1	S&S
One-Arm Dumbbell Row	1	S&S
Shoulders		
Machine Lateral Raise	2–3[1]	8–12
Barbell Overhead Press	1	S&S
Traps		
Smith Machine Shrug	1	S&S

[1] warm-up

Strength & Endurance

DAY 4 Chest, arms

EXERCISE	SETS	REPS
Chest		
Dumbbell Flye	2–3[1]	8–12
Dumbbell Press	1	S&E
Smith Machine Incline Bench Press	1	S&E
Biceps		
Dumbbell Incline Curl	2–3[1]	8–12
Standing Dumbbell Curl	1	S&E
Triceps		
Pushdown	2–3[1]	8–12
Machine Dip	1	S&E

[1] warm-up

DAY 5 Legs, abs

EXERCISE	SETS	REPS
Quads/Hams		
Leg Extension	2–3[1]	8–12
Leg Curl	2–3[1]	8–12
Leg Extension	1	S&E
Leg Curl	1	S&E
Calves		
Standing Calf Raise	1	S&E
Abs		
Machine Crunch	1	S&E

[1] warm-up

DAY 6 Back, shoulders, traps

EXERCISE	SETS	REPS
Back		
Pull-Up	2–3[1]	8–12
Close-Grip Lat Pulldown	1	S&E
Wide-Grip Seated Row	1	S&E
Shoulders		
Lateral Raise	2–3[1]	8–12
Machine Overhead Press	1	S&E
Traps		
Dumbbell Shrug	1	S&E

[1] warm-up

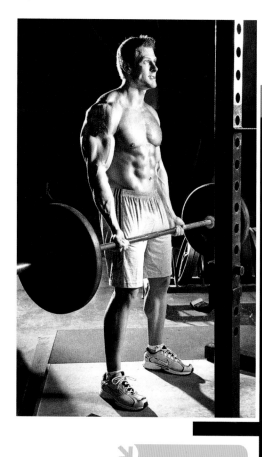

BARBELL CURL

ARM YOURSELF
Heavy curls on your strength and size days will spur new muscle growth

HIGHS & LOWS PROGRAM WEEKS 3+4

Strength & Size

DAY 1 Chest, arms

EXERCISE	SETS	REPS
Chest		
Incline Flye	2–3[1]	8–12
Cable Crossover	1	S&S
Dumbbell Incline Press	1	S&S
Smith Machine Bench Press	1	S&S
Biceps		
Preacher Curl	2–3[1]	8–12
Barbell Curl	1	S&S
Dumbbell Incline Curl	1	S&S
Triceps		
Pushdown	2–3[1]	8–12
Cable Overhead Extension	1	S&S
Close-Grip Smith Machine Bench Press	1	S&S

[1] warm-up

DAY 2 Legs, abs

EXERCISE	SETS	REPS
Quads/Hams		
Leg Extension	2–3[1]	8–12
Leg Curl	2–3[1]	8–12
Leg Extension	1	S&S
Leg Curl	1	S&S
Leg Press	1	S&S
Calves		
Standing Calf Raise	1	S&S
Abs		
Machine Crunch	1	S&S

[1] warm-up

DAY 3 Back, shoulders, traps

EXERCISE	SETS	REPS
Back		
Lat Pulldown	2–3[1]	8–12
Seated Cable Row	1	S&S
One-Arm Dumbbell Row	1	S&S
Smith Machine Bent-Over Row	1	S&S
Shoulders		
Machine Lateral Raise	2–3[1]	8–12
Dumbbell Overhead Press	1	S&S
Smith Machine Upright Row	1	S&S
Traps		
Smith Machine Shrug	1	S&S
Dumbbell Shrug	1	S&S

[1] warm-up

Strength & Endurance

DAY 4 Chest, arms

EXERCISE	SETS	REPS
Chest		
Dumbbell Flye	2–3[1]	8–12
Dumbbell Press	1	S&E
Smith Machine Decline Bench Press	1	S&E
Smith Machine Incline Bench Press	1	S&E
Biceps		
Dumbbell Incline Curl	2–3[1]	8–12
Standing Dumbbell Curl	1	S&E
Dumbbell Scott Curl	1	S&E
Triceps		
Pushdown	2–3[1]	8–12
Machine Dip	1	S&E
Rope Pushdown	1	S&E

[1] warm-up

DAY 5 Legs, abs

EXERCISE	SETS	REPS
Quads/Hams		
Leg Extension	2–3[1]	8–12
Leg Curl	2–3[1]	8–12
Leg Extension	1	S&E
Leg Curl	1	S&E
Smith Machine Squat	1	S&E
Calves		
Standing Calf Raise	1	S&E
Abs		
Machine Crunch	1	S&E

[1] warm-up

DAY 6 Back, shoulders, traps

EXERCISE	SETS	REPS
Back		
Pull-Up	2–3[1]	8–12
Close-Grip Lat Pulldown	1	S&E
Pullover	1	S&E
Standing Cable Row	1	S&E
Shoulders		
Lateral Raise	2–3[1]	8–12
Machine Overhead Press	1	S&E
Reverse Pec-Deck Flye	1	S&E
Traps		
Dumbbell Shrug	1	S&E
Shrug	1	S&E

[1] warm-up

Chapter 5

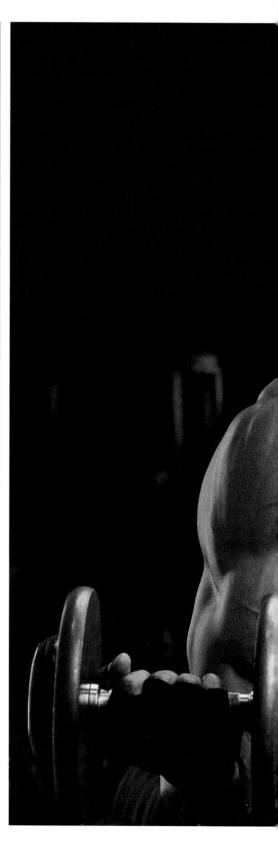

Taking Sides

Train unilaterally to topple strength plateaus while you torch your midsection

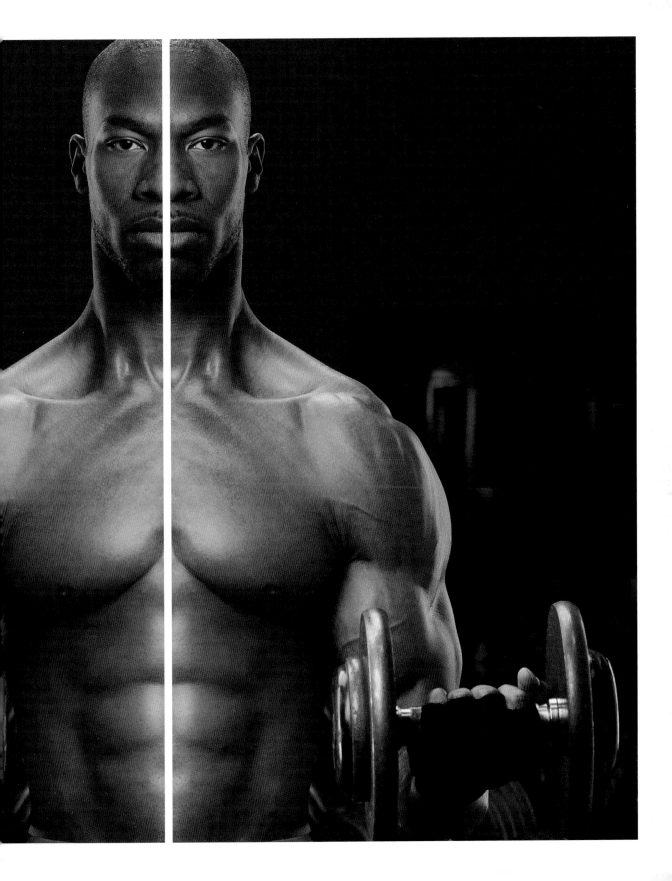

BOREDOM COULD WRECK US ALL. JUST

watch a Chekhov play: all those rheumy-eyed Russians moping around their crumbling estates, harboring unrequited love or brooding with envy. Chekhov knew it was a problematic conceit, and he took pains to right it. He said that if a gun is introduced in the first act, it had better go off by the third. Chances are, midway through the second act you're hoping everyone onstage gets a cap popped in their backsides as a motivator.

The connection may be tenuous, but training over time with little variation can cause some of the aforementioned moping and brooding. Invariably, the results are poor gains, strength plateaus and an unquenchable thirst for vodka and mail-order brides. The first two conditions can be solved with this unilateral training program. The temptation for spirits and women, however, are immune to most everything... except more spirits and women.

KEEPIN' IT FRESH

Walter Norton Jr., who's not Russian but a good French-Canadian from North Andover, Massachusetts, is particularly sharp in the keep-it-fresh school of training. A former strength and conditioning coach with the Boston Celtics and founder of the Institute of Performance and Fitness, his success is predicated on getting results for his clients, who are sometimes high school athletes and sometimes Celtics star Paul Pierce.

Unilateral training — training one side of your body at a time to shore up strength imbalances and concentrate all your effort on the target muscle — is fundamental to Norton's philosophy. The key to success isn't necessarily wholesale change, in which everything you've done in the past is buried in an unspecified location and most of your gym time is spent doing handstand push-ups on a vibrating plate while holding a kettlebell in your mouth (though there are some benefits to that). For our purposes, the changes will be variations of recognizable themes. The main focus is to hammer one side of the body at a time, which will produce bilateral gains in hypertrophy and strength, especially if you've been on the same page for a while.

"This program is a perfect complement to what you're already doing, and it's a great way to get past training plateaus if you've been doing the same things again and again," Norton explains. "You'll stress the muscles in slightly different ways and identify bilateral differences. On top of that, you'll strengthen your torso."

MORE STIMULI

Norton says a common problem with many athletes and gym rats is the "strong limbs, weak torso" disease. By training unilaterally, you'll learn firsthand how bad you've got it. The real driver of the program, however, are the gains incited by this focused approach. Change for the sake of change oversimplifies the Muscle Confusion Principle, but if you're a seasoned trainee, change for the sake of change keeps you in the gym and invested in the process, both mentally and physically. "The more

THE UNILATERAL WORKOUT

This program, created by Walter Norton Jr., is designed to supplement an existing routine. The exercises are paired and should be performed at the beginning and/or end of a typical training day, as indicated. The workouts are separated into two phases, each of which should be used for 2–3 weeks at a time for best results. Paired workouts for legs, upper body and biceps/triceps contain exercises that cover multiple muscle groups. (Shoulders don't have their own day because they're stressed so much in the other upper-body routines.) If you prefer to focus on specific muscles, feel free to mix and match these exercises according to your training needs.

stimuli you give your muscles and mind, the better they respond," he states.

For Norton, unilateral training isn't just a means to an end. He says it more accurately reflects the stresses and demands of everyday life such as the bending and reaching movements he considers unilateral in nature. When possible, he avoids having clients lie down or sit in a machine to push resistance. "I just don't think the body is meant to train that way," he remarks.

Some moves in this program are quite advanced, and others will torch your midsection as well as the target muscle. Done consistently and with proper form, this workout will replace any notion of boredom with thoughts of pain. Consider it a cap in your ass.

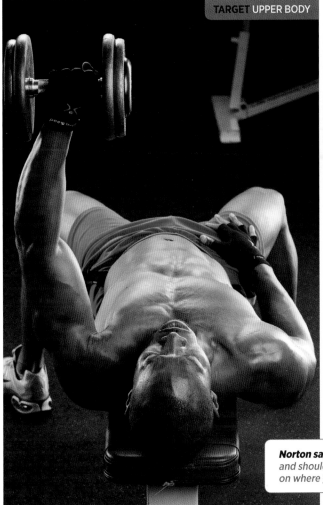

TARGET UPPER BODY

← FLAT-BENCH DUMBBELL PRESS

Lie faceup on a flat bench with your feet flat on the floor, grasping a dumbbell in one hand at the bottom of a press. Keeping your core tight, press the weight up and squeeze your pec, then return to the start position. Repeat for reps, then switch sides.

Variation:
DUMBBELL INCLINE PRESS CIRCUIT

Adjust an incline bench to 30–45 degrees and sit with your back squarely against the bench, feet flat on the floor, dumbbells in hand. Press one weight up for four reps, then repeat with the other arm. Without resting, press both dumbbells to full-arm extension and do four reps with one arm while keeping the other arm extended. Repeat with the other arm. Without resting, return both weights to the start position and do four bilateral reps to finish the circuit.

Norton says: "This is a great way to warm up the chest and shoulders or completely burn them out, depending on where you place the exercise in your routine."

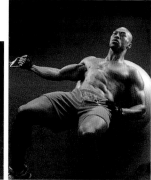

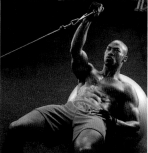

TARGET UPPER BODY

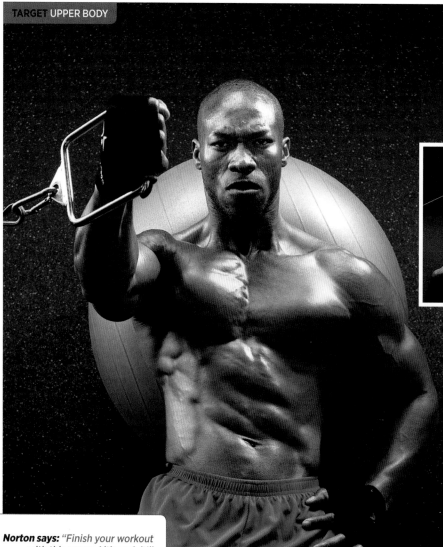

← EXERCISE-BALL ONE-ARM CABLE FLYE

Lie faceup on an exercise ball with your feet on the floor, knees bent and back fully supported so you're parallel to a low-pulley cable station. Making sure there's no slack in the cable, grasp the handle with your near hand. Keeping your elbow bent slightly and your arm moving in the same plane as your shoulder, bring your hand directly over your chest. Squeeze your pec at the top, then slowly return to the start while maintaining your posture and stability through the torso and glutes. Alternatively, you could use a dumbbell. Repeat for reps, then switch sides.

Norton says: *"Finish your workout with this move. Although it'll isolate and torture your pecs, the core requirement is significant, so expect to feel it in your midsection. This and the dumbbell row from the floor may be all the abdominal training you need to do for the day."*

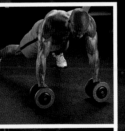

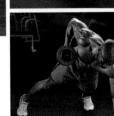

> **Norton says:** *"Done with proper form, this exercise is as difficult as any you'll find. Your shoulders play a huge role."*

ALTERNATE-GRIP CHIN (Not shown)

Grasp a fixed overhead bar using a wide grip, one palm facing you and the other facing away; wrap your thumbs around the bar. Hang freely with your arms fully extended, knees bent and ankles crossed behind you. Contract your lats to raise your chin past the bar, concentrating on keeping your elbows out and pulling them down to your sides. Hold the peak-contracted position momentarily before lowering to the start position. Alternate your grip each set.

Norton says: *"Most of your upper body will feel this one, especially your grip, shoulders and torso. The size and strength of your back will improve as well. Add weight when you can complete four sets of six reps."*

↑ DUMBBELL ROW FROM THE FLOOR

With your feet a little wider than shoulder width, get into the top position of a push-up and grasp two dumbbells placed on the floor so your hands are aligned with your shoulders. Pull one dumbbell toward the same-side hip, then return it to the floor. Repeat with the opposite arm. Don't let your hips drop or your feet come off the floor. As you progress, bring your feet closer together and perform all reps for one side before switching.

PHASE 1

EXERCISE	SETS	REPS	TIMING
Alternate-Grip Chin	4	6	start of workout
Dumbbell Incline Press Circuit	3	12[1]	start of workout

[1] each side

PHASE 2

EXERCISE	SETS	REPS	TIMING
Exercise-Ball One-Arm Cable Flye	3	15[1]	end of workout
Dumbbell Row From the Floor	3	4[1]	end of workout

[1] each side

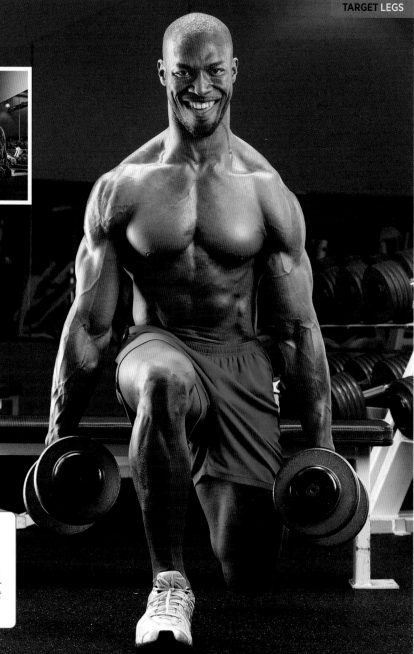

TARGET LEGS

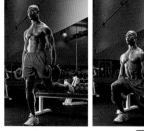

ONE-LEG SQUAT →

Stand erect facing away from a flat bench with a light dumbbell in each hand. Extend your left leg behind you and place the top of your foot on the bench. Your knee will form about a 90-degree angle. Begin by bending your right knee and hip as if to sit in a chair until your quad is parallel to the floor. Your right knee should be directly over your ankle and shouldn't internally rotate. Return to standing by driving your heel into the floor. Repeat for reps, then switch legs.

Norton says: *"This is one of the single best exercises for leg strength, development and real-life activities. Start your workout with this movement. It's a whole-body move, and one that'll boost your heart rate."*

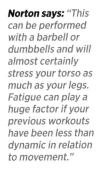

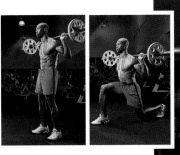

WALKING LUNGE →

Stand erect holding a barbell across your upper back, then take a long stride forward with one foot. Bend both knees to descend toward the floor, making sure your front knee doesn't pass your toes. Stop just short of your trailing knee touching down. Push up by driving through the heel of your front foot and bring your back leg forward to meet your front leg. Keep your core tight. Switch legs and repeat.

Norton says: *"This can be performed with a barbell or dumbbells and will almost certainly stress your torso as much as your legs. Fatigue can play a huge factor if your previous workouts have been less than dynamic in relation to movement."*

Norton says: *"This move is hard to perform well. You can gauge your improvement based on how smooth the exercise feels over time. Everything should contribute evenly: Your torso, quads, hips, shoulders and forearms should all work together."*

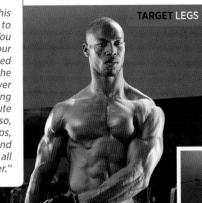

← ONE-ARM, TWO-LEG ROTATIONAL ROW (ADVANCED MOVE)

Stand erect and alongside a low-pulley cable station with your right foot closest to it. Grasp the handle in your left hand so your arm crosses your body. Turn your torso to face the pulley and bend both your knees and hips into a squat. Loading your front (right) leg, drive your foot into the floor as you extend your knees and hips to return to standing, rotating your hips away from the pulley to face the opposite direction as you pull the handle toward your right hip. Your body will move up and down during the exercise but shouldn't lean right or left. In the top position you should be on the ball of your right foot and standing erect. Repeat for reps, then switch sides.

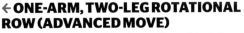

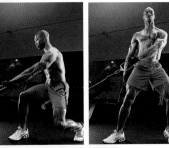

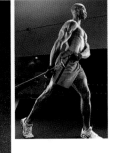

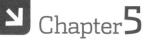
TARGET LEGS

EXERCISE-BALL LEG CURL, 2 IN 1 OUT
(Not shown)

Lie faceup on the floor with your legs extended and your calves atop an exercise ball. With your arms flat on the floor, raise your hips and torso to form a straight line from feet to shoulders. Flex your hamstrings to curl the ball toward your glutes for a two-count, then roll the ball out with one leg, pull it back in and roll it out with the other. Imagine you're trying to crush the ball with each leg.

Norton Says: *"This may guarantee a hamstring cramp the first time out, but it'll shape your hams and strengthen your glutes to no end. Add four reps (two per leg) each week."*

ONE-LEG ECCENTRIC LEG PRESS
(Not shown)

Sit in a leg-press machine and place your feet shoulder-width apart on the sled. Keep your chest up and lower back pressed into the backpad. Unlock the safeties and, using only one leg, bend your knee to slowly lower the sled, focusing on the eccentric portion of the move. Stop before your glute lifts off the pad, then push up explosively to the top position. Squeeze your leg hard. Repeat for reps, then switch sides.

Norton Says: *"Use this movement as a finisher. Start at eight reps with a slow negative rep (eight seconds) followed by an explosive push to the start. Change up the reps, sets or duration of the eccentric rep as desired. Add two reps each week."*

PHASE 1

EXERCISE	SETS	REPS	TIMING
One-Leg Squat	3	6[1]	start of workout
Exercise-Ball Leg Curl, 2 In 1 Out	3	4[1]	start of workout

[1] each side

PHASE 2

EXERCISE	SETS	REPS	TIMING
Walking Lunge	3	8[1]	end of workout
One-Leg Eccentric Leg Press	3	8[1]	end of workout
One-Arm, Two-Leg Rotational Row[2]	3	8[1]	start of workout

[1] each side   [2] advanced move

TARGET BICEPS & TRICEPS

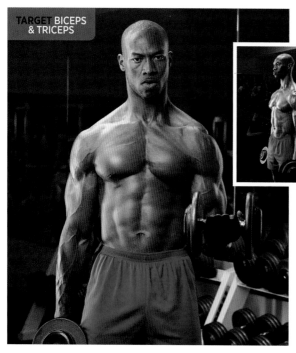

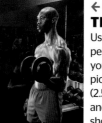

← ONE-ARM "DOWN THE RACK" CURL

Using a mirror or partner, do perfect palms-forward curls until your form is compromised, then pick up the next lightest dumbbell (2.5-pound increments work best) and repeat. No hip swing or elbow shortage, just great technique until the muscle is exhausted. Do this six times to failure with each level of resistance, then switch sides.

Norton Says: *"Finish up arm day with this killer. Choose six dumbbells in descending order, 2.5-pound increments, and move from one to the next without rest. A partner who calls you out when your form breaks down is helpful, as is a truthful eye in the mirror."*

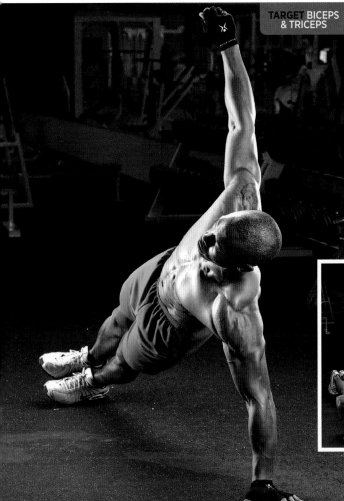

TARGET BICEPS & TRICEPS

← PUSH-UP WITH ROTATION

Get into the bottom position of a push-up, chest touching the floor. Explode up into a side plank, rotating your hips so they're perpendicular to the floor and both arms are straight, one in the air and the other bearing all your weight, feet stacked. Return to the start and repeat on the opposite side. For those who become advanced quickly, do 10 reps per side before switching.

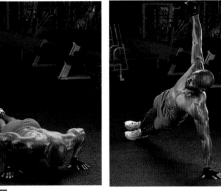

Norton Says: *"A good way to awaken the entire upper body and shoulder complex is with this twist on the push-up. It can also be the final blow to fatigued triceps, chest and torso muscles, as they must all work together to produce great form. Add two reps (one per side) each week."*

ONE-ARM DOUBLE-ROPE PRESSDOWN (Not shown)

Stand erect in front of a high-pulley cable and grasp both parts of the rope attachment with one hand using a neutral grip. With your knees bent slightly, lean forward a bit at the waist and pin your elbow at your side. Flex your triceps and press the rope toward the floor until your arm is fully extended. Squeeze and hold for a brief count before returning to the start. Repeat for reps, then switch sides.

Norton Says: *"Add this at the end of your workout to fatigue your triceps and grip strength completely. Hold the ropes at the midpoint."*

ALTERNATE DUMBBELL INCLINE

PHASE 1

EXERCISE	SETS	REPS	TIMING
One-Arm Double-Rope Pushdown	3	12–15[1]	end of workout
Alternate Dumbbell Incline Curl	3	10[1]	end of workout

[1] each side

PHASE 2

EXERCISE	SETS	REPS	TIMING
Push-Up with Rotation	3	8[1]	start/end of workout
One-Arm "Down the Rack" Curl	6	to failure	end of workout

[1] each side

Chapter 6

Chain of Command

Redefine chain training by using these new techniques to stimulate massive muscle growth

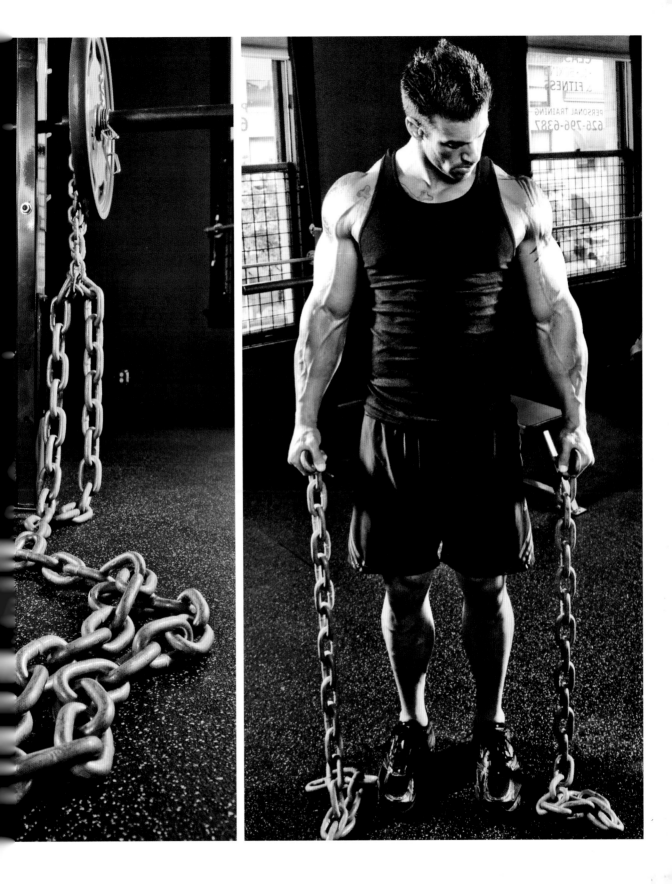

WHEN YOU SEE CHAINS HANGING FROM a barbell, it's safe to assume there's a powerlifter lurking nearby with visions of strength and explosiveness dancing in his head. Yet chains aren't solely the province of the powerlifting set. Used correctly, they're a simple and effective tool for stimulating muscle growth. If you've ever been jealous of the guys you've seen lugging buckets of chains into the gym, wishing you could get in on their "hardcore" motif, this workout offers you a whole new way to reap the myriad benefits of lifting with chains without having to shave your head and grow some neck rolls. Chains add a unique drag to the barbell known as linear variable resistance. Picture a set of chains attached to either end of a bar. At the bottom of a squat, the chains are piled on the floor. As you stand up, they lift off the floor link by link, forcing you to move an increasing amount of weight. This makes you recruit more fast-twitch muscle fibers — the ones that contract the fastest and strongest, and grow the biggest.

Linear variable resistance is effective because the weight becomes heavier during the second half of the range of motion (ROM), where you're stronger. When you use a barbell alone, you're limited by how much you can lift during the first part of the movement (when you're weakest). Some muscle groups — the bi's and delts in particular — don't fully kick in until you're nearly halfway through the rep. During a curl, for example, the load you can lift through the first half isn't enough to overload your biceps at the top. Using

CHAIN LATERAL RAISE →

The first 30 degrees of the ROM involves primarily the supraspinatus. The deltoids don't contribute until after this point, which is when the chains add weight.

Setup: Attach a D-handle to a small (3/8") adjustment chain, and attach that to the end of a large chain. The first link of the large chain should lift off the floor when your arms hang at your sides. When you can do more than 15 reps lifting one link at a time, attach the adjustment chain to the middle link of the large chain to lift two links at a time.

Execution: Raise your arms out to your sides in an arc until they're parallel to the floor. Pause at the top, then slowly return along the same path to the start.

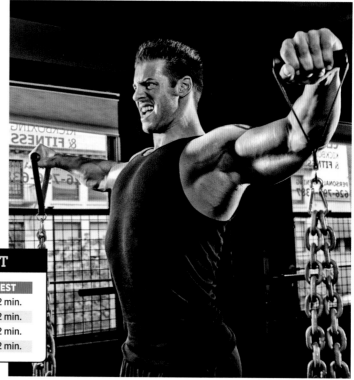

SAMPLE SHOULDER WORKOUT

EXERCISE	SETS/REPS	REST
Dumbbell Overhead Press	3/8–10	1–2 min.
Dumbbell Upright Row	3/8–12	1–2 min.
Chain Lateral Raise	3/10–15	1–2 min.
Bent-Over Lateral Raise	3/12–15	1–2 min.

chains solves this problem.

You can also use chains to target specific areas of various muscle groups. Research shows that during a squat, for example, the vastus medialis (the teardrop just above the inner knee) is engaged during the top half of the exercise. Since this is where you're strongest, a bar isn't enough to overload the muscle. But adding chains to the mix increases the weight at the right time to target the teardrop and stimulate growth.

Try the following moves on for size, incorporating them into your usual routines as shown in our sample workouts.

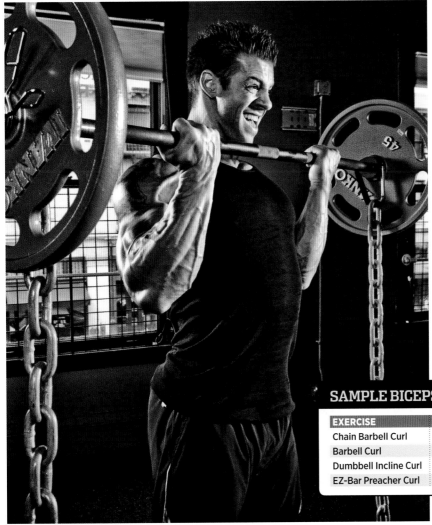

← CHAIN BARBELL CURL

Using chains overloads the biceps during the top half of the move.

Setup: Attach the end of a large (5/8") chain to a carabiner and slide it onto the end of a bar as if to load a plate. Find a weight that challenges you for three sets of 8-12 reps. At first, the chains may provide sufficient resistance.

Execution: Stand erect with your feet shoulder-width apart, grasping the bar with an underhand grip. Curl the weight toward your chest, keeping your elbows fixed at your sides. Pause at the top, then slowly return to the start position.

SAMPLE BICEPS WORKOUT

EXERCISE	SETS/REPS	REST
Chain Barbell Curl	3/8–12	1–2 min.
Barbell Curl	2/8–12	1–2 min.
Dumbbell Incline Curl	3/10–12	1–2 min.
EZ-Bar Preacher Curl	3/12–15	1–2 min.

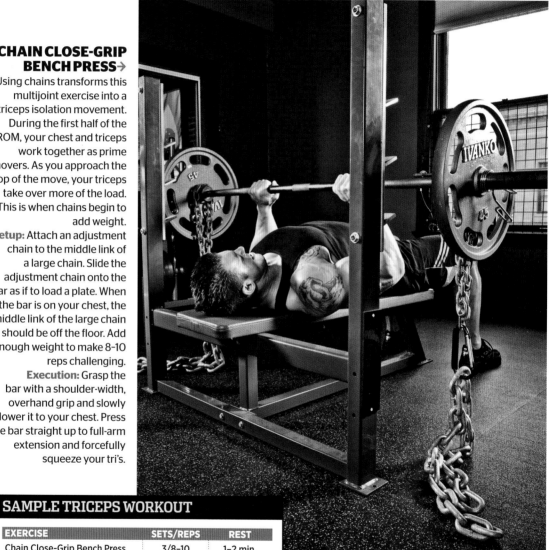

CHAIN CLOSE-GRIP BENCH PRESS→

Using chains transforms this multijoint exercise into a triceps isolation movement. During the first half of the ROM, your chest and triceps work together as prime movers. As you approach the top of the move, your triceps take over more of the load. This is when chains begin to add weight.

Setup: Attach an adjustment chain to the middle link of a large chain. Slide the adjustment chain onto the bar as if to load a plate. When the bar is on your chest, the middle link of the large chain should be off the floor. Add enough weight to make 8-10 reps challenging.

Execution: Grasp the bar with a shoulder-width, overhand grip and slowly lower it to your chest. Press the bar straight up to full-arm extension and forcefully squeeze your tri's.

SAMPLE TRICEPS WORKOUT

EXERCISE	SETS/REPS	REST
Chain Close-Grip Bench Press	3/8–10	1–2 min.
Close-Grip Bench Press	2/8–10	1–2 min.
Lying Triceps Extension	3/8–12	1–2 min.
Pushdown	3/12–15	1–2 min.

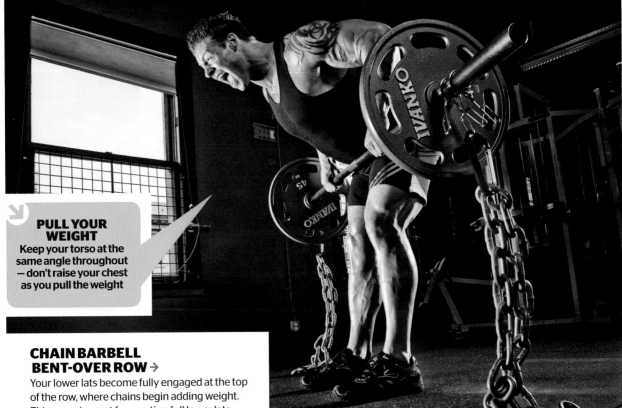

CHAIN BARBELL BENT-OVER ROW →

Your lower lats become fully engaged at the top of the row, where chains begin adding weight. This move is great for creating full lower lats that jut straight out from your torso, adding dramatic width to your back.

Setup: Attach the middle link of a large chain to a carabiner, and attach that to the end of a spring collar positioned toward the end of a bar. This prevents the chains from piling up under the weight plates. Load the bar with enough weight to make 6–10 reps challenging.

Execution: Grasp the bar with a shoulder-width grip and lean forward at the hips until your torso is nearly parallel to the floor. Pull the bar into your midsection, then slowly lower it to full-arm extension.

SAMPLE BACK WORKOUT

EXERCISE	SETS/REPS	REST
Chain Barbell Bent-Over Row	3/6–10	1–2 min.
Barbell Row	3/6–10	1–2 min.
Wide-Grip Lat Pulldown	3/8–10	1–2 min.
Straight-Arm Pulldown	3/12–15	1–2 min.

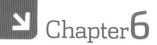
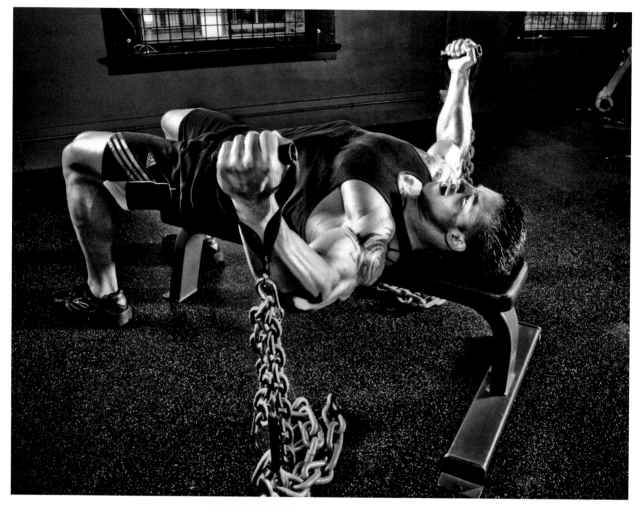

CHAINFLYE↑

Using chains on flyes better overloads the inner pecs, which engage as your hands come together, and reduces the amount of weight you hold at the bottom of the move. This allows a better stretch at the beginning without placing excessive stress on your shoulder joints.

Setup: Attach a D-handle to an adjustment chain, and attach that to the middle link of a large chain. The first link on the large chain should be off the floor at the bottom of the flye. If you can do more than 15 reps with a heavy chain, use two large chains.

Execution: Lie faceup on a flat bench, grasping the handles above your chest. Keeping your elbows bent slightly, slowly lower your arms out to your sides in an arc, then reverse the motion. This exercise can also be performed on an incline or decline bench.

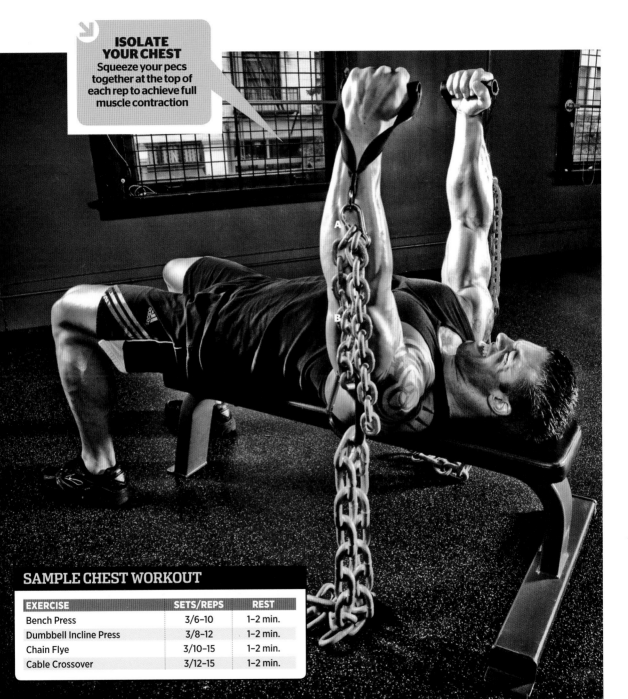

ISOLATE YOUR CHEST
Squeeze your pecs together at the top of each rep to achieve full muscle contraction

SAMPLE CHEST WORKOUT

EXERCISE	SETS/REPS	REST
Bench Press	3/6–10	1–2 min.
Dumbbell Incline Press	3/8–12	1–2 min.
Chain Flye	3/10–15	1–2 min.
Cable Crossover	3/12–15	1–2 min.

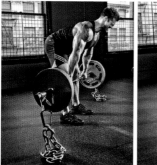
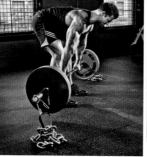

CHAIN ROMANIAN DEADLIFT →

Using chains on this move will better target your glutes, the major players in squats and conventional deadlifts. **Setup:** Attach the middle link of a large chain to a carabiner, then attach that to the end of a spring collar positioned toward the end of a bar. This prevents the chains from piling up under the weight plates. Load the bar with enough weight to make 6–10 reps challenging. **Execution:** Stand erect with your feet about shoulder-width apart and bend your knees slightly. Grasp the bar with a shoulder-width grip and slowly lower it to about mid-shin, then push your hips forward until you're standing upright. Keep your lower back arched throughout the movement.

SAMPLE HAMSTRING WORKOUT

EXERCISE	SETS/REPS	REST
Chain Romanian Deadlift	3/6–10	1–2 min.
Romanian Deadlift	2/6–10	1–2 min.
Lying Leg Curl	3/10–15	1–2 min.

SAMPLE QUAD WORKOUT

EXERCISE	SETS/REPS	REST
Chain Squat	3/6–10	1–2 min.
Front Squat	3/8–12	1–2 min.
Leg Press	3/8–12	1–2 min.
Leg Extension	3/12–15	1–2 min.

ADDING CHAINS TO YOUR TRAINING WILL BUILD TONS OF STRENGTH

CHAIN IT UP

There are many other chain moves you can try in addition to the exercises in this article. Here's a list of alternatives to consider.

MUSCLE GROUP	EXERCISE	TARGET MUSCLE
Chest	Chain Bench Press	Inner pecs
Shoulders	Chain Barbell Overhead Press	Middle deltoids
Back	Chain One-Arm Dumbbell Row	Lower lats
Biceps	Chain "Dumbbell" Curl	Biceps
Triceps	Chain Kickback	Lateral triceps heads
Quads	Chain Step-Up	Vastus medialis
Traps	Chain Shrug	Upper traps

Chapter 7

More Power to You

Power training isn't just for athletes anymore. Blast your body with this explosive routine that boosts strength and size

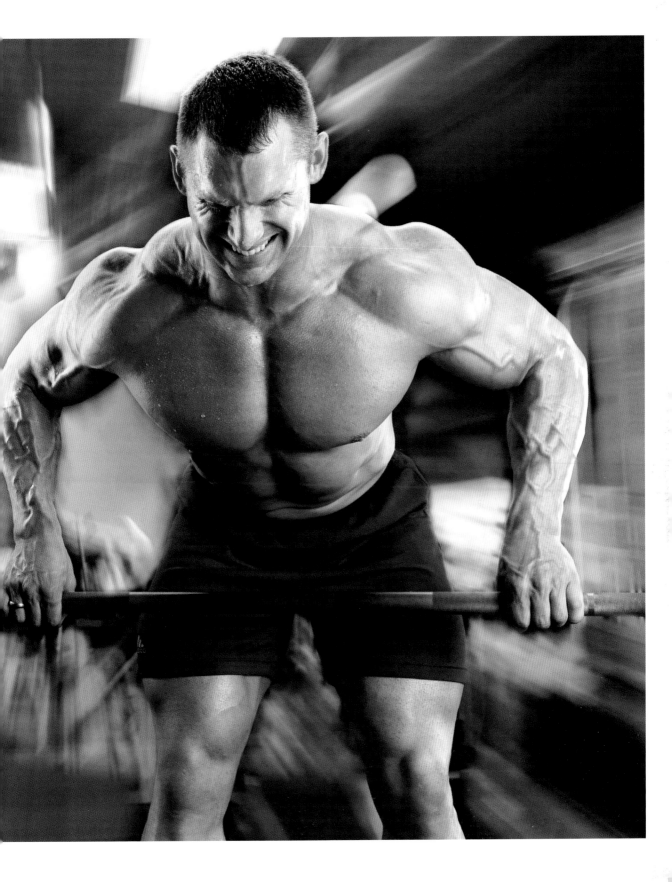

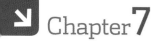
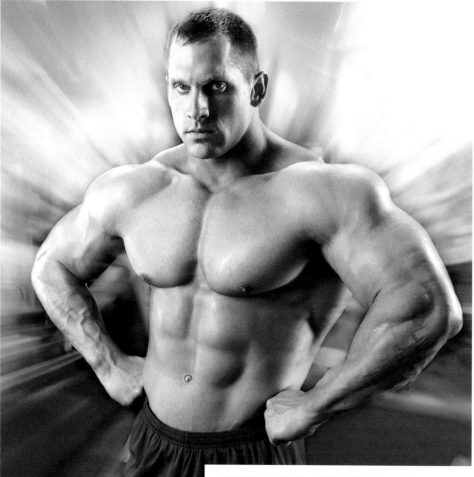

THINK OF POWER AS EXPLOSIVENESS: A-ROD TURNING

on a waist-high fastball, Floyd Mayweather blasting some poor schmuck with a right hand, Adrian Peterson bursting through a weak-side hole. Power is all about how much energy you can generate in the shortest period. For nonathletes mainly interested in building muscle or getting ripped, spending precious gym time trying to become the MVP of your weekend pickup game might not sound all that appealing. But becoming more powerful doesn't happen in a vacuum.

"Power and strength go hand in hand," says Mike McGuigan, PhD, professor of exercise physiology at Edith Cowan University (Australia) and member of the MUSCLE & FITNESS Advisory Board. "Power is produced by the combina-

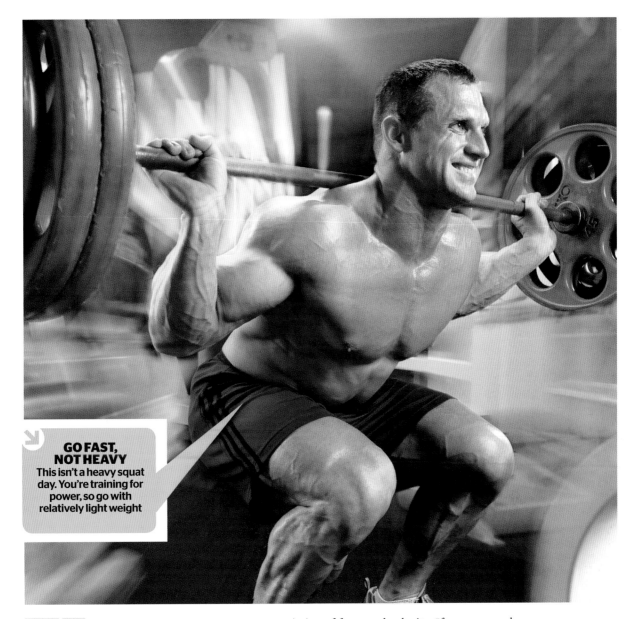

If you can produce more force, you'll become more powerful. Studies show that the more powerful you are, the stronger you are, and vice versa

tion of force and velocity. If you can produce more force, you'll become more powerful. And a lot of studies now show that the more powerful you are, the stronger you are, and vice versa." In other words, building power also means increasing strength, which in turn means adding mass. It's all so beautifully intertwined.

Power training, however, has its own set of rules and regulations. Contrary to the visceral idea of explosiveness, a power-building routine doesn't involve lifting ungodly poundages. For the most part,

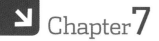
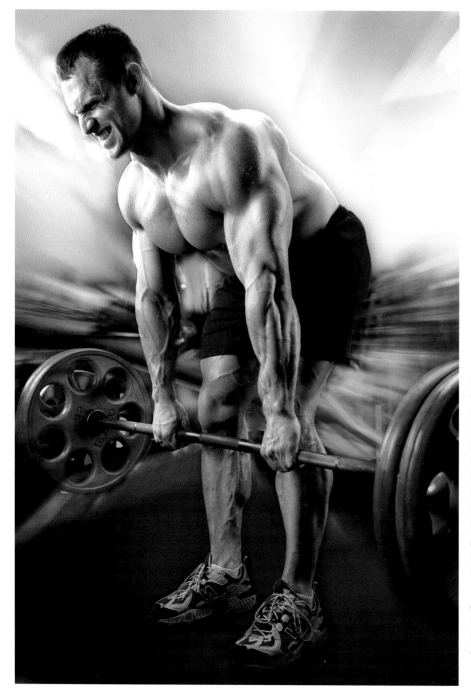

It's not just the amount of weight or how quickly you move the weight, but it's the intent to move the weight quickly that greatly increases your power

lighter weights dominate. "Research has shown that it's not necessarily the amount of weight or how fast you move the weight, but it's the intent to move the weight quickly that can increase your power," McGuigan explains. "So trying to lift heavy loads explosively can be a good strategy for increasing power along with strength."

He adds that using a variety of exercises — or a mixed-methods approach that involves resistance training with 30%–50% of your one-

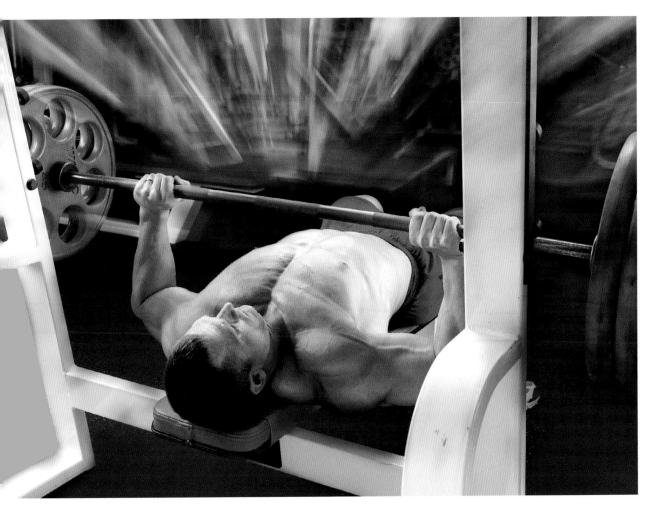

rep maximum, plyometrics such as jumps and unweighted bounds, and ballistic-type movements such as jump squats and medicine-ball throws — appears to produce the best results.

Energy levels are equally important during these workouts. McGuigan says research indicates that power is sensitive to fatigue and that athletes who first complete a heavy training phase score considerably lower on power measurements afterward. Use rest periods of 2–4 minutes between sets, which will involve lower-than-usual reps themselves. Remember: To enhance power, you need to generate as much of it as you can on each and every rep.

Don't see the advantage of altering your workouts to add power training, especially since you have no interest in blowing through a weak-side hole? Hear out McGuigan one last time: "A big advantage of this type of training is that it's not typically something your body is used to, so it can be a good way to shock it into getting bigger and stronger." Enough said.

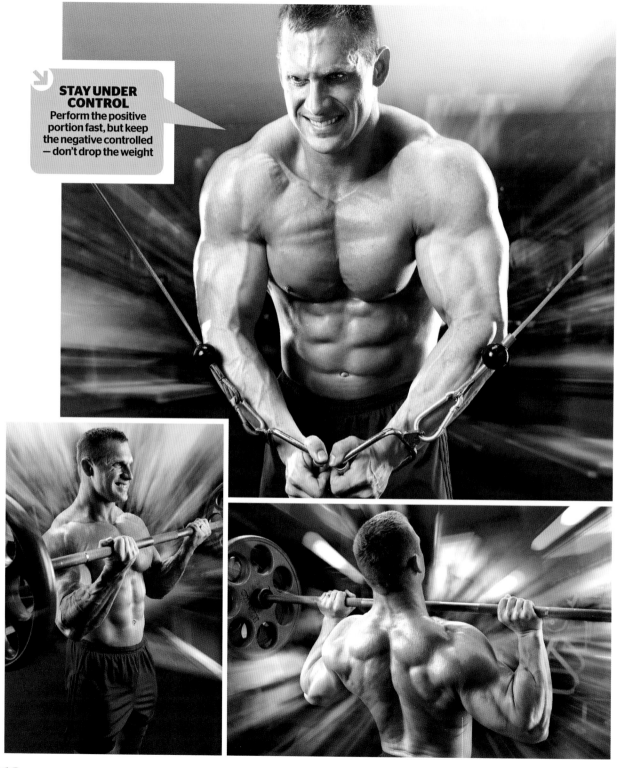

THE POWER TRAINING WORKOUT

WORKOUT 1 MONDAY

MUSCLE GROUP	EXERCISE	SETS	REPS[1]	REST
Chest	Bench Press	4	8,5,6,12	2 min.
	Dumbbell Incline Press	4	8,5,6,12	2 min.
	Dumbbell Flye	4	8,5,6,12	2 min.
	Cable Crossover	4	8,5,6,12	2 min.
Triceps	Close-Grip Bench Press	4	8,5,6,12	2 min.
	Dip	4	8,5,6,12	2 min.
	Lying Triceps Extension	4	8,5,6,12	2 min.
Abs	Do your typical workout.			

WORKOUT 2 TUESDAY

MUSCLE GROUP	EXERCISE	SETS	REPS[1]	REST
Legs	Squat	4	8,5,6,12	2 min.
	Leg Press	4	8,5,6,12	2 min.
	Leg Extension	4	8,5,6,12	2 min.
	Romanian Deadlift	4	8,5,6,12	2 min.
Calves	Standing Calf Raise	4	8,5,6,12	2 min.
	Seated Calf Raise	4	8,5,6,12	2 min.

WORKOUT 3 THURSDAY

MUSCLE GROUP	EXERCISE	SETS	REPS[1]	REST
Shoulders	Barbell Overhead Press	4	8,5,6,12	2 min.
	Smith Machine Upright Row	4	8,5,6,12	2 min.
	Lateral Raise	4	8,5,6,12	2 min.
	Bent-Over Lateral Raise	4	8,5,6,12	2 min.
Traps	Barbell Shrug	4	8,5,6,12	2 min.
Abs	Do your typical workout.			

WORKOUT 4 FRIDAY

MUSCLE GROUP	EXERCISE	SETS	REPS[1]	REST
Back	Barbell Row	4	8,5,6,12	2 min.
	Wide-Grip Lat Pulldown	4	8,5,6,12	2 min.
	Reverse-Grip Lat Pulldown	4	8,5,6,12	2 min.
	Seated Cable Row	4	8,5,6,12	2 min.
Biceps	Barbell Curl	4	8,5,6,12	2 min.
	Dumbbell Incline Curl	4	8,5,6,12	2 min.
	Preacher Curl	4	8,5,6,12	2 min.
Forearms	Barbell Reverse Curl	4	8,5,6,12	2 min.
	Barbell Wrist Curl	4	8,5,6,12	2 min.

[1] On Set 1, use a weight with which you can normally do up to 30 reps or more (yes, ridiculously light!). On Set 2, use a weight with which you can normally do 15–20 reps. For these two sets, move quickly and explosively on the positive rep and slowly on the negative. On Set 3, use a weight that limits you to six reps, working as fast and explosively as possible. On Set 4, use a weight that limits you to 12 reps; after reaching failure, immediately reduce the weight by about 30% and do as many reps as possible to failure. Use a slow, controlled pace.

THE POWER PYRAMID PROGRAM

Pyramid training is a popular protocol employed by almost every type of weight-trainer, from recreational lifters to strongman competitors. Typically you'd change the resistance on each successive set by following a pattern of ascending or descending sets, but here we combine them to create what's known as triangle pyramid training: You start light and go heavier on the next two sets, then your fourth set is lighter.

We modify the program further by varying the rep speed. On the first set use a weight that would allow you to get 30 reps or more on that exercise, but do only eight reps. (You don't want to fatigue your muscles when training for power; the fatiguing sets will come later.) Perform these eight reps as quickly and as explosively as possible on the positive portion, then go slow and controlled on the negative. This will serve as both a warm-up and a power-building set.

On your second set, use a weight that would allow you to get 15–20 reps. Stop at five reps, but perform them as quickly and explosively as possible on the positive portion, and slow and controlled on the negative.

On the third set you increase the weight again, this time to something that allows you to get only six reps. Perform as many reps as you can; you should reach failure at or around the sixth rep. Try to work as fast and as explosively as possible. Remember, just trying to move a heavy weight explosively can increase power. This set will serve as both a power and strength set. It's also the peak of the pyramid, and now you begin the descent.

Your last set is actually two sets in one. Choose a weight that allows you to complete about 12 reps, then try to reach failure as close to that number as possible. At failure, immediately reduce the weight by about 30% and continue doing as many reps as you can to failure. Called a drop set, this is technically two sets performed back to back. Rest only as long as it takes you to change the weight. Perform all your reps at a slow and controlled pace — two seconds on the

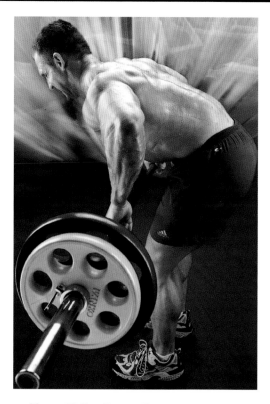

positive and 2–3 on the negative.

The combination of ascending sets, descending sets and change in rep speed produces a program that develops power, strength and mass. Our sample workout follows a four-day training split, so you can train on any four days of the week that fit your schedule. This pyramid scheme can also be incorporated right into your existing program. Simply do the number of reps with the weight we suggest for each of four sets for each exercise you normally do. Whether you follow our plan or adapt it to your current regimen, stick with it for a minimum of four weeks and a maximum of six.

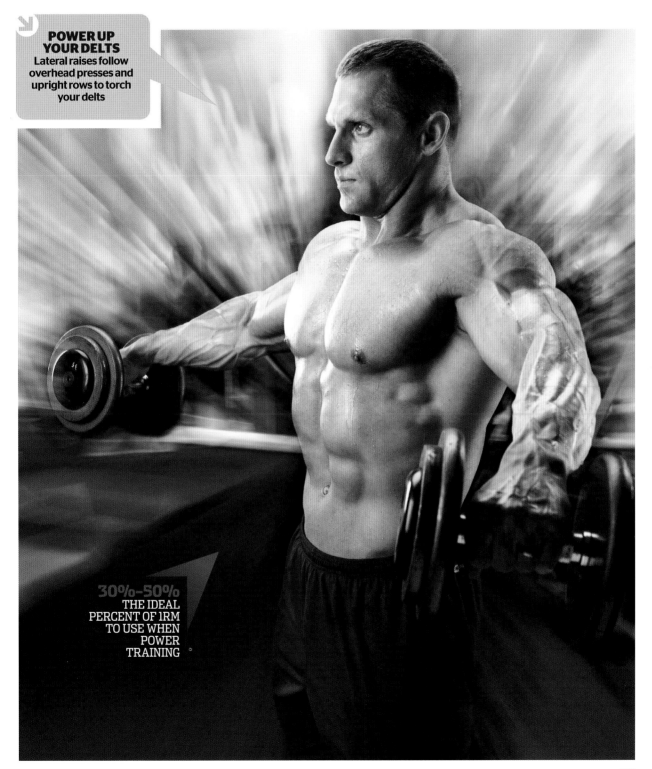

30%–50%
THE IDEAL PERCENT OF 1RM TO USE WHEN POWER TRAINING

Chapter 8

Achtung, Baby!

German Volume Training and its 10x10 set-and-rep scheme will take you to the brink of failure, then build you back up again bigger and stronger than before

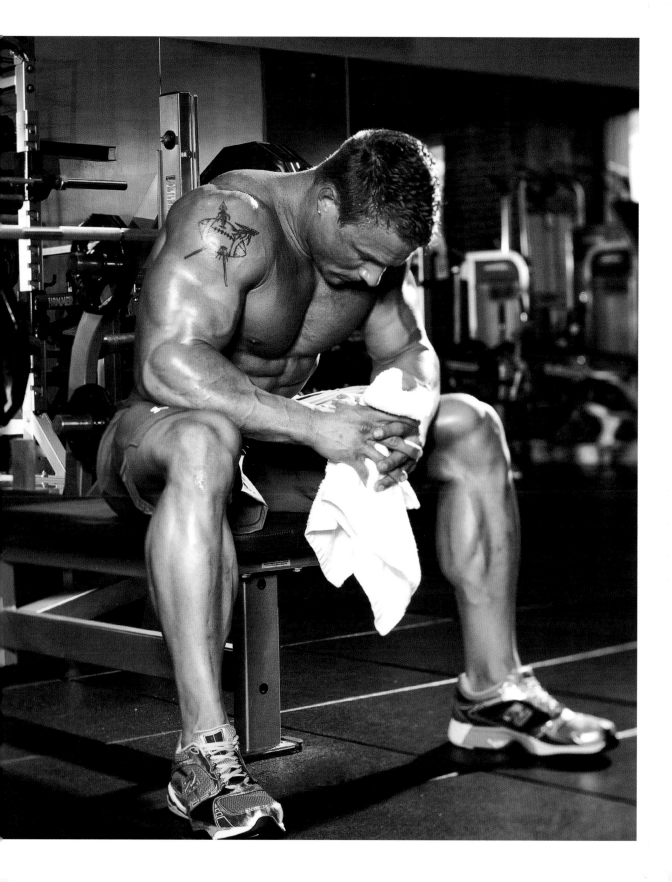

THE GERMANS ALWAYS MAKE good stuff. From beer and cars to pharmaceuticals and superabsorbent chamois towels, you'll find evidence of superior Teutonic manufacturing everywhere you look. German Volume Training (GVT), the country's signature weight-training program, is no exception.

Mechanical precision and simplicity have historically been hallmarks of German production, and these characteristics are reflected in the exacting nature of GVT. For four weeks, you'll perform 10 sets of 10 reps of one exercise for most bodyparts — a simple proposition on paper, but one that'll challenge you like nothing you've ever done in the gym.

This proven torture test has been used for decades by the world's best bodybuilders and weightlifters to pack on size in a short period. So hoist your stein, don your lederhosen and pretend it's Oktoberfest, because you're about to learn how to get after it the German way.

GVT will challenge you like nothing else. This proven torture test has been used for decades by the best bodybuilders and weightlifters to pack on size in a short period

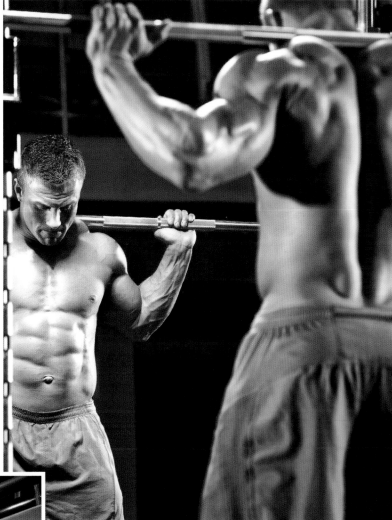

← THE ARCHITECT

In the 1970s, German Olympic weightlifting coach Rolf Feser wanted to design an early-season training program that would add lean mass. Feser knew that to handle Olympic-level weight totals in the clean and jerk and the snatch, his team needed to first increase the muscular cross section necessary for the production of force. The best way he found to do this was with an introductory cycle of simple, high-volume hypertrophy work.

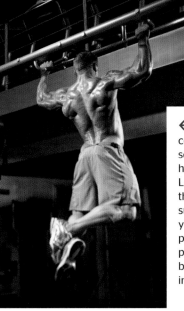

← If 10 sets of 10 conventional pull-ups seems daunting, you have a few options: Loop a band around the bar and use it to support one foot, use your gym's assisted pull-up machine or put both feet on a bench and perform inverted rows.

↑ HUGE LIKE A HUN

Ten sets of 10 reps. With any exercise, that kind of volume's going to hurt. Stick it out, though, because volume adds size like nothing else can. Since GVT targets a single muscle group repeatedly with the same movement pattern, it forces that bodypart to adapt to the monumental stress you're putting on it. Your muscles will adapt by growing, because that's what they have to do to handle the extra load. In the case of GVT, that load is so intense and directly targeted that it shocks the adaptation process into warp speed, mandating hypertrophy in a very short time.

Chapter 8

GVT EQUALS INTENSITY
Be prepared to feel an intense muscle burn before diving into this program

THE WORKOUT

DAY 1: Quads, Hamstrings, Calves, Abs

EXERCISE	SETS	REPS	REST
Back Squat	10	10	60 sec.
Leg Curl	10	10	60 sec.
Seated Calf Raise	10	10	60 sec.
Incline Sit-Up	3	15	60 sec.

DAY 2: Chest, Back

EXERCISE	SETS	REPS	REST
Bench Press	10	10	60 sec.
Pull-Up	10	10	60 sec.
Cable Crossover	3	10	60 sec.
Seated Row	3	1	60 sec.

DAY 3: Off

DAY 4: Triceps, Biceps, Shoulders

EXERCISE	SETS	REPS	REST
Dip	10	10	60 sec.
EZ-Bar Curl	10	10	60 sec.
Shrug	3	10	60 sec.
Leaning Bent-Over/ Lateral/Front Raise[1]	3	8	90 sec.

DAYS 5–7: Off

[1] Stand erect next to a fixed object you can grasp at about chest level, move your feet as close to its base as you can and lean to the side so your nonworking arm is fully extended. Beginning with the dumbbell behind your back using a neutral grip, raise it out to your side until your elbow is at shoulder level, then return to the start. Move the weight to your hip and execute the movement the same way. Lastly, move the dumbbell so your palm faces your quad, then raise it to eye level. That's one rep.

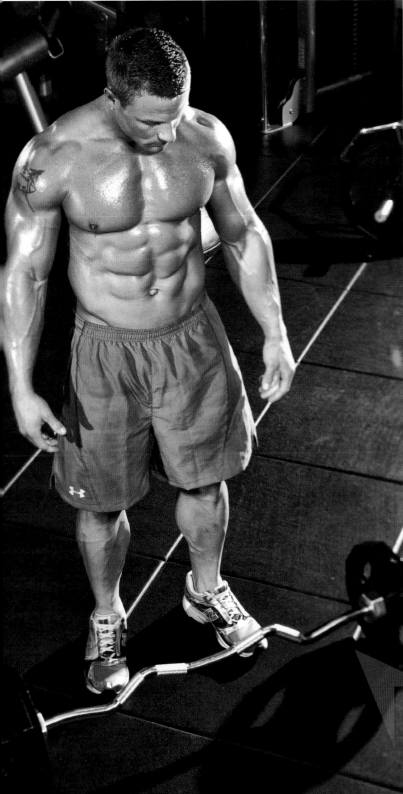

← GVT: HOW IT SHOULD FEEL

For each 10x10 exercise, start with 60% of your one-rep max, or use a weight with which you can perform 20 reps. Put some serious thought into this, because your success with this initial selection is how you'll gauge your progress over the next four weeks. Here's how a typical progression should feel:

> **Sets 1–3** The weight is too light. The reps come easily. This feels more like a French workout. You're having doubts.

> **Sets 4–5** A tremor in your system. Pain makes an entrance. You can still make it to 10, but you're entering a lactic environment and your muscles begin to burn.

> **Sets 6–7** This is definitely not as easy as you had thought. In fact, on your seventh set you can barely squeeze out six reps. Your muscles are on fire, and you're cursing everyone who ever told you that getting a pump was supposed to feel good.

> **Sets 8–9** Oddly, you're somehow able to mount a comeback here and get in 10 reps on both sets. When you experience this rebound effect, you're on the right track. Your central nervous system is adapting to the movement. Ride the wave.

> **Set 10** Thirty more seconds to glory. Dig deep. Finish strong.

LIMIT REST PERIODS TO 60–90 SECONDS BETWEEN SETS

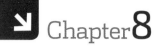
**BUILD
BIG GUNS**
Doing 10 sets of 10 reps
on curls will give your
biceps a massive pump
to spur new growth

← MECHANICAL PRECISION

Since you'll perform one exercise
per bodypart, selecting the best
overall movement for each is
crucial. For chest and legs, this
means compound multijoint lifts
such as the bench press and back
squat, supplemented with lighter-
volume exercises for supporting
muscle groups such as the delts
and abs to maintain balance.

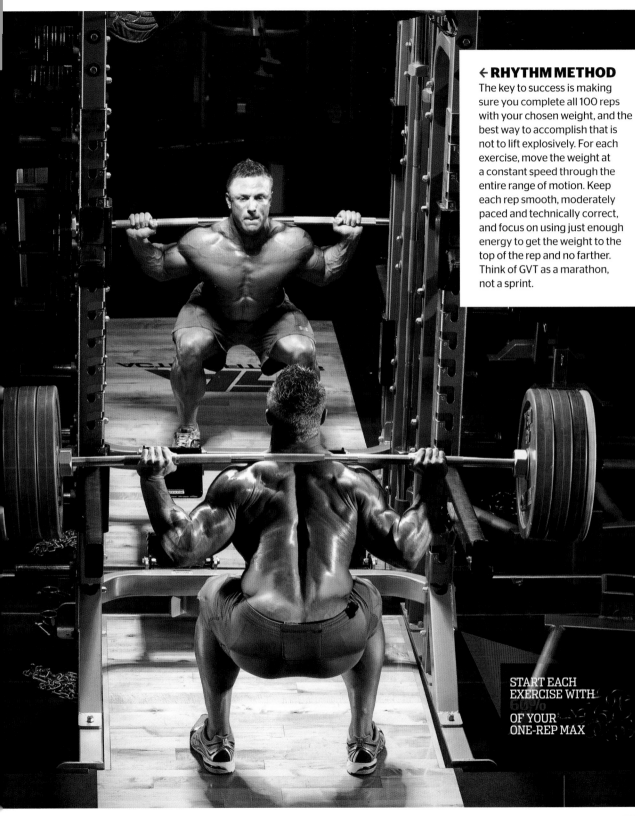

←RHYTHM METHOD

The key to success is making sure you complete all 100 reps with your chosen weight, and the best way to accomplish that is not to lift explosively. For each exercise, move the weight at a constant speed through the entire range of motion. Keep each rep smooth, moderately paced and technically correct, and focus on using just enough energy to get the weight to the top of the rep and no farther. Think of GVT as a marathon, not a sprint.

START EACH EXERCISE WITH 60% **OF YOUR ONE-REP MAX**

BIG MOVES, BIG REPS
Compound exercises like the barbell bench press will help you get the most out of GVT

CYCLE IT →

After four weeks, you're going to be sore. Very, very sore. Performing just one exercise per bodypart and working repetitively in the same plane also puts you at significant risk of overtaxing your joints. For these reasons, along with the mental break you'll need after four weeks of 10x10, GVT isn't a program you want to follow year-round.

NO TIME FOR WIENERSCHNITZEL →

You'll need a stopwatch to perform this program properly, and you must limit your rest between sets to 60–90 seconds. These short rest intervals are how you accrue the cumulative fatigue that makes GVT feel so "good" during those brutal sixth and seventh sets. They also hasten the adaptation process and build your mental toughness by preventing you from giving in to the temptation to lengthen your rest periods when things get dicey.

Chapter 9

The 5/3/1 Phenomenon

Personalize your workouts like a pro with one of the Internet's most popular programs

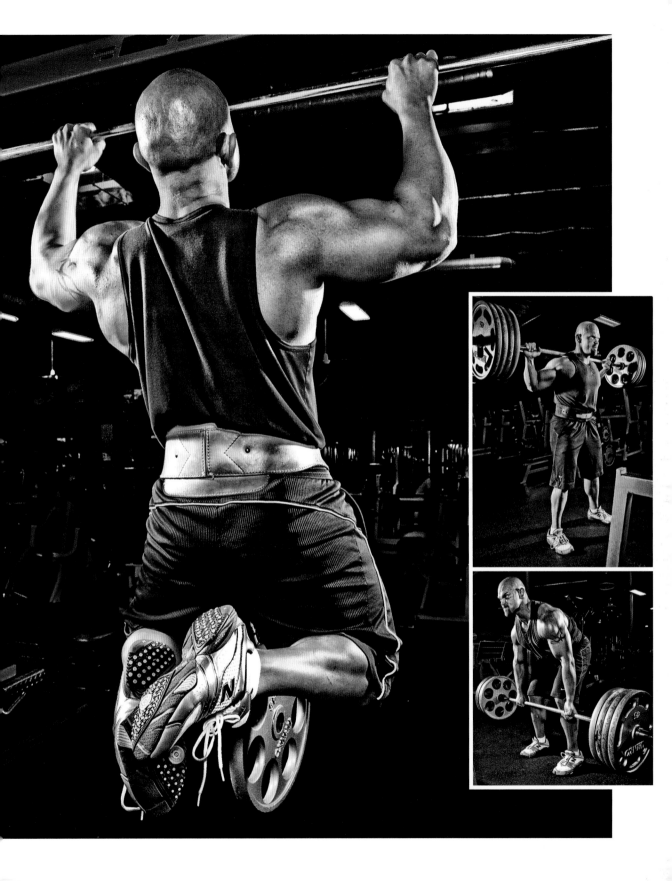

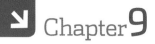

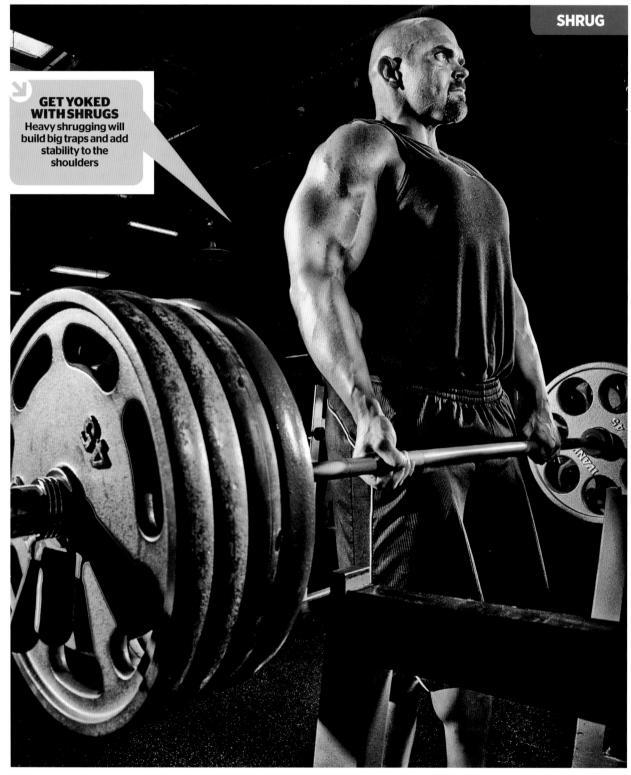

SHRUG

GET YOKED WITH SHRUGS
Heavy shrugging will build big traps and add stability to the shoulders

WE ALL HAVE A TRAINING ARSENAL AT our disposal. It consists of our equipment, capabilities, ideas and knowledge. When we know what we want, we break out our weaponry and take dead aim at whatever athletic target we're looking to hit. The idea is to strive for better accuracy, which means knowing what you need to get the job done. You want to use what you've got in an organized, coherent way so you make progress week after week.

Enter Jim Wendler's 5/3/1 program. The director of strength and development at Elite Fitness Systems in London, Ohio, and former starting fullback at the University of Arizona (Tucson), Wendler is uniquely qualified to create a program that's adaptable across the spectrum of strength disciplines. As an elite powerlifter with a 1,000-pound squat to his credit, he knows a thing or two about getting strong. Ten years of consulting with strength coaches, athletes and gym owners from all over the world has helped him form some definitive conclusions on what lifters need in terms of programming, exercise selection and equipment.

According to Wendler, 5/3/1 is more than a program, template and set-and-rep scheme: It's a new way to think about your arsenal. It's a way to break out your weapons with confidence and know exactly how to apply what you've got. It takes what we already know — exercises with which we're already familiar — and teaches us a better way to put everything together.

"This program is all about training economy," Wendler explains. "Everything you do supports your four main lifts: bench press, deadlift, military press and squat, or whatever else you choose to do. Building your program around these lifts instead of doing endless sets per bodypart gets you in and out of the gym in less than an hour with better results."

Since the introduction of the program in March 2009, people have taken notice, especially online, where it has merited "Internet sensation" status. The official 5/3/1 e-book has sold tens of thousands of copies on the Elite Fitness Systems website — the only legal means of procuring a copy. Multiple Facebook pages are devoted to it, and numerous college and high school athletic teams have adopted it as their primary lifting program.

5/3/1 gives you a set of parameters so you can design your own program and emphasize what's important to you. "When you're training for strength and size, bench presses, deadlifts and squats are essential. But with 5/3/1 you choose exercises that work the muscles that support these movements," says Matt McGorry, a trainer at New York City's Peak Performance. "That's why this program is ideal for anyone looking to add overall size or strengthen lagging muscle groups."

EVERYTHING STARTS WITH BIG MULTI-JOINT MOVES. You can choose whichever compound movements you like, but the program recommends constructing your weekly workouts around the bench press, deadlift, military press and

5/3/1 SAMPLE REP-MAX PROGRESSION

WEEK 1

EXERCISE	IRM	WORKING MAX
Bench Press	200 pounds	180 pounds
Squat	300 pounds	270 pounds
Deadlift	325 pounds	292.5 pounds

WEEK 5

EXERCISE	ORIGINAL WORKING MAX	NEW WORKING MAX (90% 1RM)
Bench Press	180 pounds	185 pounds
Squat	270 pounds	280 pounds
Deadlift	292.5 pounds	302.5 pounds
Rep-Max Calculator: Weight x Reps x .0333 + Weight = Estimated 1RM		

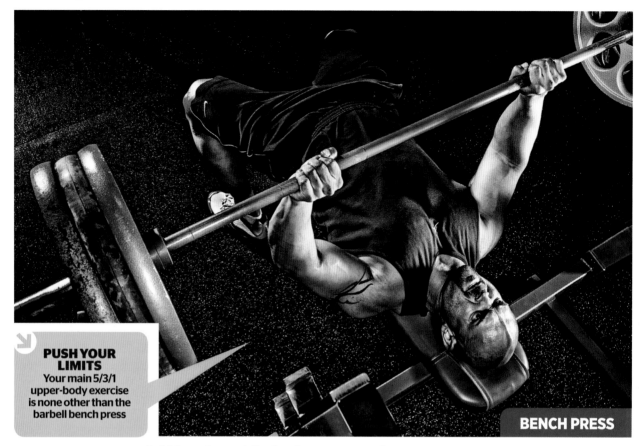

BENCH PRESS

squat — none of which require specialized equipment or fancy machines. "These are the most efficient exercises for building size and strength," Wendler says. "This isn't a secret, but everyone acts like it is."

Next, you begin and work almost exclusively with weights that are 60%–85% of your one-rep max. Using submaximal loads has several advantages: You won't kill yourself in the gym every day, which will help you recover faster, and you'll eliminate the anxiety of handling heavy weights every session. "When I ask someone how much he can bench, the answer is always more than he realistically can," Wendler points out. "When you take a step back like this, you know you're working with weights you can actually handle."

Everything you do in the weight room has a cumulative effect. Using lighter weights on your main lifts vs. working up to one big set accumulates tonnage, which is the aggregate total of everything you move in the gym. The more tonnage you accrue over time, the bigger and stronger you get.

"You need enough stimulus to get stronger, but you don't want to go overboard," Wendler notes. "Your body is like a car. If you press the accelerator to the floor all day, every day, the engine is going to burn out. That's exactly what most people do in the weight room."

The third major 5/3/1 principle is the notion of slow, steady progress. Instead of ramping things up quickly and trying to blast through your sticking points, 5/3/1 increases training volume a little at a time, making improvements manageable and consistent. Your body adapts to weight increases over a four-week period, allowing you to progress slowly and surely before you move on. These month-to-month increases may not seem like much until you've added 50–60 pounds to all your main lifts in a year's time.

"[The typical method of switching] training programs every few weeks guarantees you won't learn enough about your body to optimally design a routine for yourself," McGorry says. "This program provides a solid line of improvement that'll give you the proper feedback and let you know where you stand."

Finally, you're encouraged to compete against yourself and break personal records every time you're in the gym. On your last set of every main exercise, perform as many reps as you can at a given percentage. Then plug the weight and number of reps into a rep-max calculator and compare your results to what you did in previous weeks. This gives you a definitive goal for each workout.

5/3/1 IS A PRECISE PERCENTAGE-BASED SYSTEM, so you'll need to know your one-rep maxes for your 3–4 main lifts before you get started. If you train alone and don't feel safe attempting a one-rep max, do as many reps as you can with a weight you can lift for 8–10 reps. Then plug your results into the rep-max calculator: Weight x Reps x .0333 + Weight = Estimated 1RM.

Once you establish your numbers, multiply each 1RM by 90%. This is your working max, and you'll use it

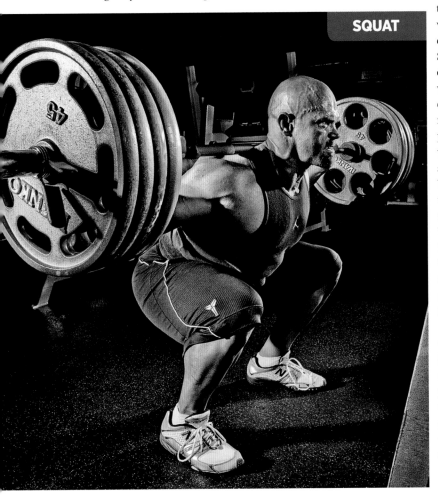

SQUAT

to derive the percentages of weight you'll train with in your daily workouts. (See "5/3/1 Sample Rep-Max Progression" on page 85.) For your 5/3/1 working sets, you'll use 65%–95% of your working max, or 60%–85% of your 1RM, progressively increasing the weight on each of your three sets. You do five reps per set in Week 1 and three in Week 2, then pyramid down from five reps to three reps to one rep in Week 3. (See "5/3/1 Sample Training Split" on page 89.) Wendler suggests starting with an empty bar, then repping out using 30%–40% of your working max until you're used to it.

Remember, these numbers are percentages of your working max, not your 1RM. If a percentage of your working max yields an odd number, round up or down depending on how you feel. Week 4 is a deload week, when you reduce the intensity and give yourself a break after

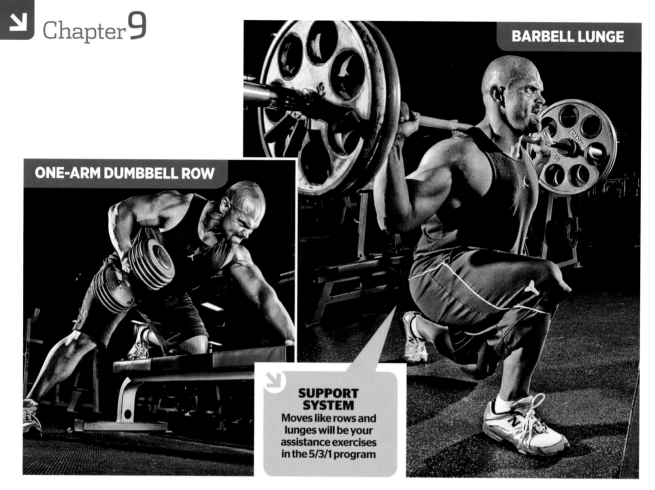

BARBELL LUNGE

ONE-ARM DUMBBELL ROW

↘ **SUPPORT SYSTEM**
Moves like rows and lunges will be your assistance exercises in the 5/3/1 program

three weeks of climbing the percentage ladder.

There's a final caveat, and it's what makes 5/3/1 special. For the last main set each week — using 85%, 90% and 95% of your working max, respectively — the split lists corresponding sets of five reps, three reps and one rep. These, however, are only the minimum requirements. Do as many reps as you can, then plug the weight you used and the number of reps you performed into the rep-max calculator.

"You're forced to be objective about your training because you record your sessions and chart your progress," McGorry says. "After awhile, you'll notice patterns and spot trends in your programming that'll help you break records and move forward."

Once you complete a full four-week cycle, add 10 pounds to your lower-body working maxes and 5 pounds to your upper-body working maxes. Use these new numbers to calculate the next month's percentages. (See "5/3/1 Sample Rep-Max Progression.")

THE EXERCISES THAT FOLLOW YOUR MAIN LIFTS are your assistance work, and this is where 5/3/1 is adaptable to your needs. You can choose assistance moves to strengthen weak points, support your main lifts, build muscle mass or any combination of these. The options are limitless.

Wendler suggests sticking with the basics here, which means doing primarily barbell and dumbbell lifts, and eschewing machines. "You want to do exercises that give you the best transfer to the main lifts," he says. "This will get you in and out of the weight room in less time because when you do movements such as dips and chins, you hit your chest, shoulders, triceps, upper back, grip and biceps in just two exercises. What else do you need to do after that?"

Structure your assistance work according to your needs. If your lower-back strength is a limiting factor in your squat, add good mornings or hyperextensions to your routine. If your goal is to put on mass, do your assistance moves bodybuilder-style: Use higher rep ranges (10-plus) for the bodyparts you think are lagging.

Pay attention to which exercises improve your main lifts and which ones don't. If something's working, keep it in your rotation until you stop making progress, then try something else. You'll need to perform assistance moves for at least two cycles — eight weeks — before judging their efficacy, but it's important to constantly re-evaluate the ones you select.

"But don't make assistance work too important in your template," Wendler warns. "Caring more about that than your main lifts is wrong. That kind of minutiae ends up detracting from the greater good. Just choose well-rounded exercises and work your whole body through a full range of motion, and the rest will take care of itself. You won't have any weak points."

5/3/1 SAMPLE TRAINING SPLIT

EXERCISE	SETS	REPS	REST
MONDAY			
Back Squat	5/3/1	5/3/1	2 min.
Barbell Lunge	3	6	1 min.
Incline Sit-Up	3	20	1 min.
WEDNESDAY			
Bench Press	5/3/1	5/3/1	2 min.
Dumbbell Incline Bench Press	5	10	1 min.
One-Arm Dumbbell Row	5	10	1 min.
Shrug	5	10	1 min.
FRIDAY			
Deadlift	5/3/1	5/3/1	2 min.
Good Morning	5	10	1 min.
Hanging Leg Raise	3	15	1 min.
SUNDAY			
Military Press	5/3/1	5/3/1	2 min.
Chin	5	10	1 min.
Dip	1	100[1]	1 min.
Barbell Curl	5	10	1 min.

Note: For all 5/3/1 exercises, use percentages of your working max (90% 1RM): In Week 1, do three sets: 65%x5, 75%x5 and 85%x5 or to failure. In Week 2, do three sets: 70%x3, 80%x3 and 90%x3 or to failure. In Week 3, do three sets: 75%x5, 85%x3 and 95%x1 or to failure. In Week 4 (deload), do three sets: 40%x5, 50%x5 and 60%x 5.

[1] Take as much time as you need to get 100 total reps.

The Value of Volume

Jump-start your progress and smash through sticking points with this intensive full-body blast

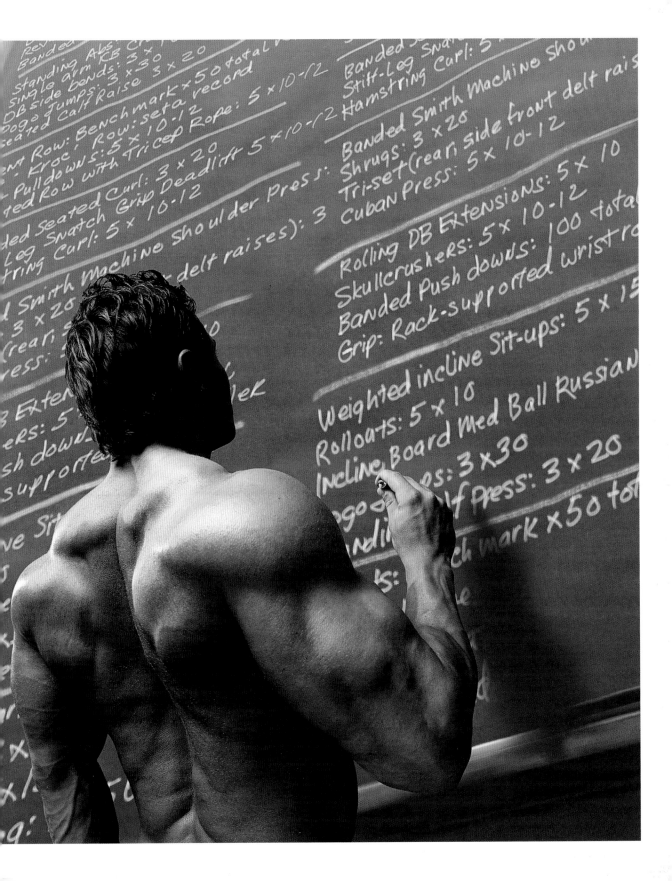

STICKING POINTS ARE LIKE

taxes. Plateaus are death. But in the weight room, as in life, you can't avoid either forever. When you've been making advances in the gym for an extended period, you're bound to come across stallouts that demand you reassess your training regimen. For most people, this entails one simple question: *Am I doing enough work?*

When this happens, the aspects of your program you should examine first are training volume — the number of sets and reps — and intensity (the weight you use for each lift compared to your one-rep maxes). When something has gone wrong, it's not always exercise selection that's the culprit; it can be the way you organize your set and rep schemes and/or the number of exercises you include.

You can add volume to a program in a variety of ways: performing additional sets per exercise or more reps in each set, adding new exercises to your routine or incorporating all three. Whatever changes you make, greater training volume means you'll work harder and longer, breaking down more muscle and forcing your body to adapt — all of which, if done correctly for a fixed period, will help you add mass and get stronger.

Boosting your training volume can improve your workout in myriad ways. First, it raises general physical preparedness (GPP) or work capacity: the amount of work you can perform in a given session (or a week or month) without fatigue being a major factor. When you raise your GPP levels, you'll recover faster from your training. Ironic, isn't it? The harder you work, the faster

POGO JUMP →

Start: Stand erect with your feet together, your knees slightly bent and your elbows bent with your hands at about chest level.
Execute: With your weight on the balls of your feet, jump up and down quickly, pushing off with only your calves. Keep your knees bent slightly.

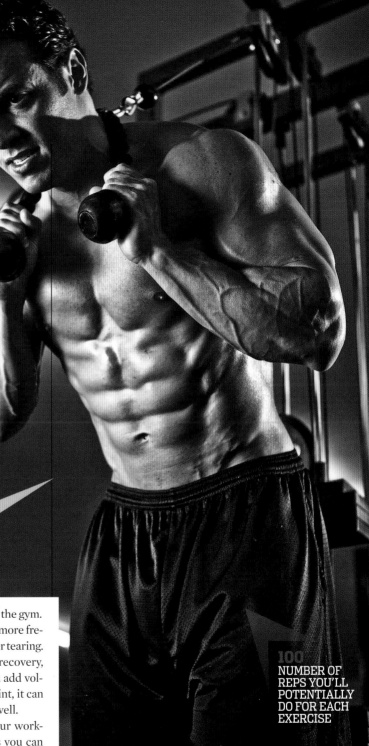

STANDING CABLE CRUNCH →

Start: Using a rope attachment at a lat pulldown station, stand erect facing away from the weight stack and grasp the rope with both hands. Pull it down around your neck so the middle of the rope touches the back of your neck.

Execute: Tighten your abs, then lean forward at the waist until your torso is past parallel to the floor.

CARVE UP YOUR ABS
This weighted midsection exercise will strengthen your core and help define your six-pack

you'll recover and the sooner you'll be back in the gym. Training with more volume will also result in more frequent and deeper microtrauma or muscle-fiber tearing. Microtraumas stimulate growth once rest, recovery, sleep and nutrition repair the muscles. If you add volume in a way that keeps your recovery on point, it can produce added muscle and strength gains as well.

Training intelligently means planning your workouts so you can train as hard and as long as you can

100
NUMBER OF REPS YOU'LL POTENTIALLY DO FOR EACH EXERCISE

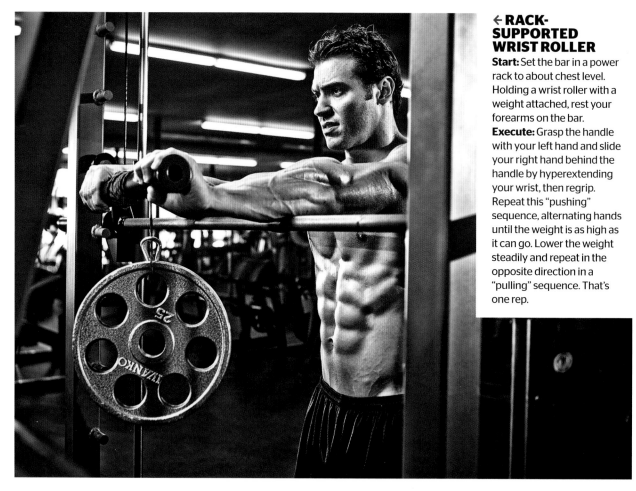

← RACK-SUPPORTED WRIST ROLLER

Start: Set the bar in a power rack to about chest level. Holding a wrist roller with a weight attached, rest your forearms on the bar. **Execute:** Grasp the handle with your left hand and slide your right hand behind the handle by hyperextending your wrist, then regrip. Repeat this "pushing" sequence, alternating hands until the weight is as high as it can go. Lower the weight steadily and repeat in the opposite direction in a "pulling" sequence. That's one rep.

without overtraining. Some people respond well to simply adding a few reps to each set or an extra exercise at the end of a gym session. Others may need to go as far as doubling their work. Just make sure not to overdo it.

"Even when you add volume, you still need to begin your workouts with compound lifts such as the bench, squat and deadlift," says Dave Cavalluzzo, strength coach and co-owner of AthElite in Hawthorne, New Jersey. "Pay attention to how increasing your volume affects these lifts, and plan your training accordingly."

How do you recognize if the extra volume is affecting your training? Track your progress in writing. If you plan to make getting bigger and stronger part of your

lifestyle, you should record your sets, reps and weight used, and constantly examine your program to detect patterns so you know what's working and what's not. When you notice something that sparks a surge in growth or strength, that's an indicator of progress.

Keeping tabs on your volume — and adjusting it based on your goals and results — is important when looking for cause-and-effect relationships in your program. Increase your training volume and if nothing happens, increase it again. If things improve, maintain that volume until you plateau, then adjust it again.

"A great way to increase volume is to ramp it up one week at a time and monitor your progress," notes John

Alvino, trainer, former competitive bodybuilder and owner of Iron Athletes in Morristown, New Jersey. "Raise your volume for three weeks, then drop it back down for a week and see how much you've progressed."

This high-volume workout features new training tools: the "total rep" concept of performing as many sets as it takes to do a fixed number of reps with a specific weight, some high-rep "finisher" exercises for arms, chest and quads, a handful of uncommon moves and two movement-based exercises that'll help stimulate significant gains in lower-body mass.

For your bench press, bent-over row and squat sets, you'll work up to a certain weight, then use that weight for your work sets; this is your benchmark weight. Take a common weight — 95, 135, 185, 225, 275, 315, etc. — and perform the exercise for the specified number of reps. As you get stronger, move to the next benchmark weight and use that for your work sets.

"Doing high-volume work on your compound lifts can kill you," Alvino warns. "So make sure to back off on those every 3–4 weeks to give your body a chance to recover."

MONDAY CHEST, BICEPS, GRIP

EXERCISE	SETS	REPS
Chest		
Bench Press (benchmark)	as needed	50
Dumbbell Butt-End Flye	5	10–12
Dumbbell Decline Press	5	10–12
Dip Finisher	as needed	50
Biceps		
Barbell Curl	5	10–12
Hammer Curl	5	10–12
Reverse Curl	5	10–12
Dumbbell-Curl Finisher	as needed	100
Grip		
Rack-Supported Wrist Roller	as needed	to failure

TUESDAY ABS, CALVES

EXERCISE	SETS	REPS
Abs		
Standing Cable Crunch	4	25
One-Arm Kettlebell Crunch	3	15 each side
Dumbbell Side Bend	3	10 each side
Calves		
Pogo Jump	3	30
Seated Calf Raise	3	20

WEDNESDAY BACK, HAMSTRINGS

EXERCISE	SETS	REPS
Back		
Bent-Over Row (benchmark)	as needed	50
Dumbbell "Kroc" Row[1]	1	to failure
Lat Pulldown	5	10–12
Seated Cable Row	5	10–12
Hamstrings		
Seated Leg Curl	3	20
Romanian Deadlift	5	10–12
Leg Curl	5	10–12

[1] A "Kroc" row is a one-arm dumbbell row where one set is performed and taken to absolute muscle failure, even if it means finishing the set with partial reps.

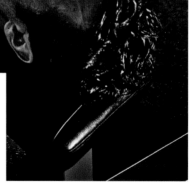

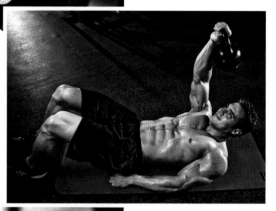

↑ ONE-ARM KETTLEBELL CRUNCH

Start: Lie faceup on the floor with your knees bent, holding a kettlebell in one hand over your face.
Execute: With the kettlebell in position, contract your abs to raise your shoulders off the floor. Repeat for reps, then switch arms.

↑ DUMBBELL BUTT-END FLYE

Start: Lie faceup on a bench holding two dumbbells above your chest using a neutral grip, elbows slightly bent.
Execute: Lower the weights out to your sides in an arc until you feel a stretch in your chest. Return along the same path while rotating your wrists so your palms face you at the top. Touch the ends together and squeeze.

HIGH-BOX SQUAT →

Start: Use a bench or a squat box that's high enough to keep your thighs a few inches above parallel when you sit on it. With a loaded barbell across your traps, stand erect facing away from the box with your feet just wider than shoulder width.

Execute: Tighten your core and descend into a squat until you touch the box, then squeeze your quads to return to standing.

PUMPED-UP VOLUME
Shortening range of motion with the high box will allow for high reps without superlight weight

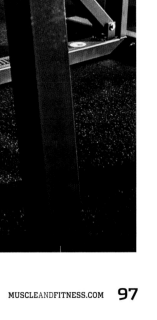

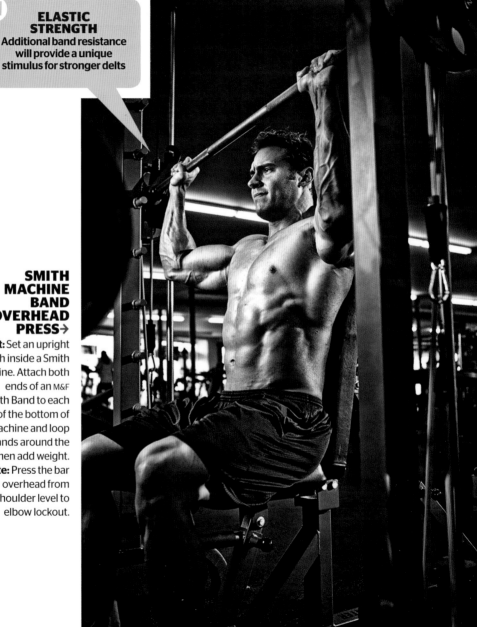

ELASTIC STRENGTH
Additional band resistance will provide a unique stimulus for stronger delts

SMITH MACHINE BAND OVERHEAD PRESS→

Start: Set an upright bench inside a Smith machine. Attach both ends of an M&F Strength Band to each side of the bottom of the machine and loop the bands around the bar, then add weight.

Execute: Press the bar overhead from shoulder level to elbow lockout.

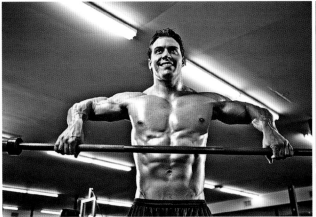
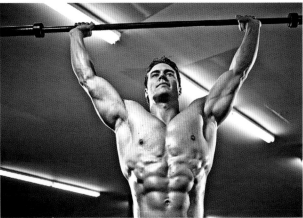

↑CUBAN PRESS

Start: Grasp a barbell with a wider than shoulder-width, overhand grip in front of your thighs.

Execute: Pull the bar up until your elbows are bent 90 degrees. Rotate your shoulders and elbows to the start of a military press. Press the bar overhead, then reverse.

THURSDAY SHOULDERS, TRICEPS, GRIP

EXERCISE	SETS	REPS
Shoulders		
Smith Machine Band Overhead Press	5	10–12
Shrug	3	20
Tri-set: Bent-Over Lateral Raise	1	8
Lateral Raise		
Front Raise		
Cuban Press	5	10–12
Triceps		
Close-Grip Bench Press	5	10
Lying Triceps Extension	5	10–12
Pushdown	as needed	100
Grip		
Rack-Supported Wrist Roller	as needed	to failure

FRIDAY ABS, CALVES

EXERCISE	SETS	REPS
Abs		
Weighted Incline Sit-Up	5	15
Rollout	5	10
Russian Twist	3	20
Calves		
Pogo Jump	3	30
Standing Calf Raise	3	20

SATURDAY QUADS

EXERCISE	SETS	REPS
Squat (benchmark)	as needed	50
Barbell Lunge	3	10–12
High-Box Squat	5	15
Backward Sled-Drag Finisher[1]	as needed	150 steps

[1] If available, drag a sled or other heavy object walking backward across an open area like a parking lot. If you don't have access to a sled, do 100 reps of leg extensions.

Chapter 11

Training for Mr. T

This high-volume multijoint workout will shoot your testosterone levels through the roof and ignite muscle growth

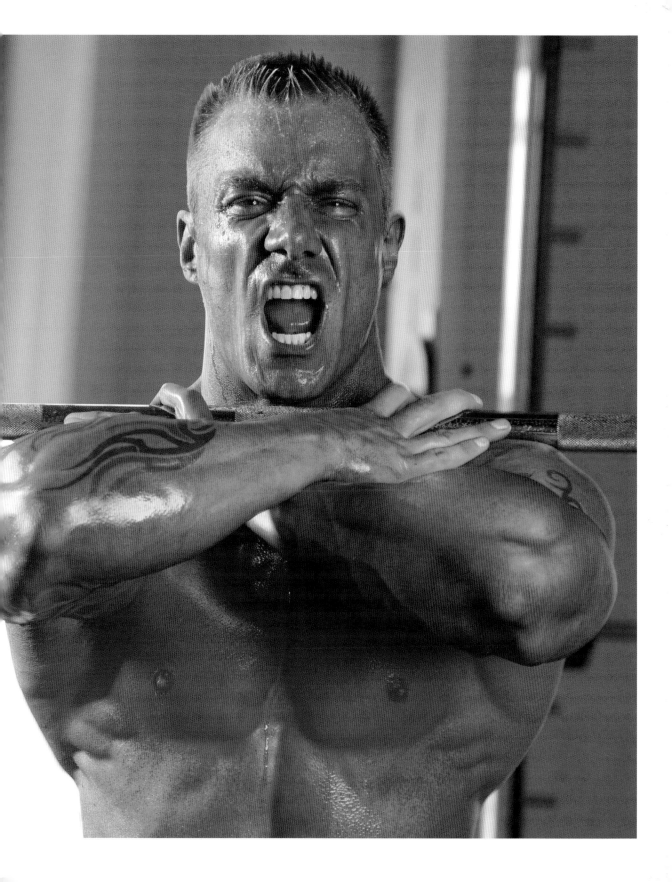

THINK OF LIFE AS A DEATH STRUGGLE with vitality. Every day you die in dribs and drabs. It may be imperceptible at first, but over time this slow leak grows until you have less of just about everything: muscle, testosterone, hair, memory, sex drive, sex appeal and sex.

Of all the subtle ways your body ages, the slowdown in testosterone production can be the most troublesome. The ultimate male hormone drives muscle growth, encourages fat loss, makes you stronger, keeps you aggressive and competitive, and fuels your libidinal blitzkriegs. Obviously, keeping your T tank topped off has its advantages, but you have to work to reap them.

Fortunately, this condition isn't like going blind or your appendix bursting. Testosterone levels drop naturally as you age, and they can be brought back up naturally — with the proper sweat equity — which is important if you want to maximize mass gain.

The science is relatively simple. Testosterone boosts muscle growth by entering muscle cells and binding to androgen receptors. Once bound, this testosterone-receptor complex enters the nuclei of the cell and activates genes that increase muscle growth. Research from the University of Connecticut (Storrs) shows that the boost in testosterone you get during workouts immediately increases the muscles' levels of androgen receptors. So, the more testosterone and androgen receptors there are, the more likely you are to stimulate growth. The key is knowing which type of workout best drives testosterone levels higher.

Again, science provides the answer. Studies show that testosterone levels rise most rapidly when you train heavy with lots of sets, target multiple muscle groups with multijoint exercises and employ short rest periods (about one minute) between sets.

To simplify the process further, we've not only given you a test-raising workout but also explained — with graphs — how and why you should follow our advice. Consider this program your hormone-replacement therapy. You won't just feel younger, you'll train that way, too.

THE FIVE GOLDEN RULES FOR GETTING BIG AND MANLY

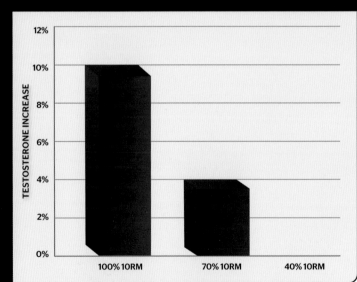

→ RULE 1
TRAIN HEAVY
This doesn't mean you should give yourself aneurysms lifting extreme loads on each set, but you also won't spend much time hoisting light weight for high reps. Research shows that when subjects trained using their 10-rep max (10RM), they experienced a 10% increase in testosterone levels. Yet when they trained with just 70% of their 10RMs — or 40% done with fast and explosive reps — they experienced little or no change in T levels.

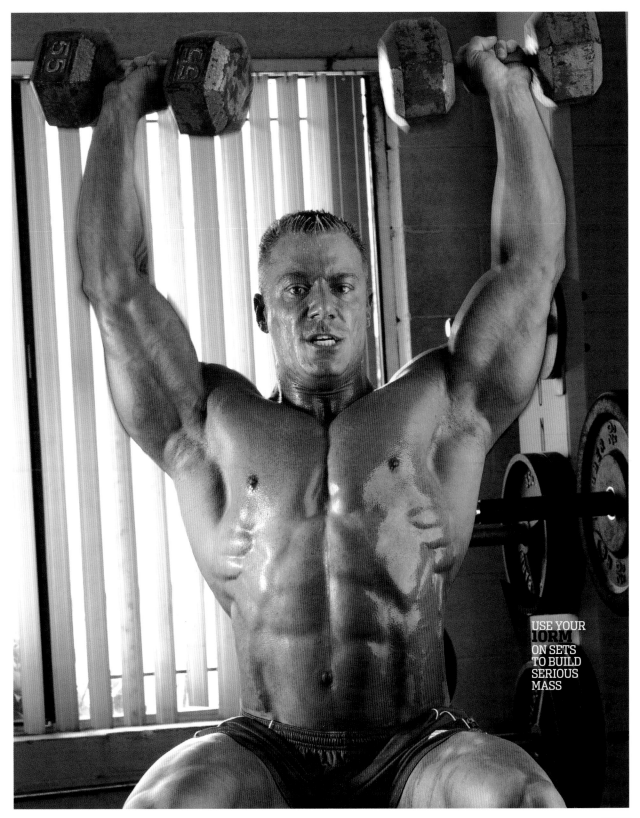

USE YOUR
1ORM
ON SETS
TO BUILD
SERIOUS
MASS

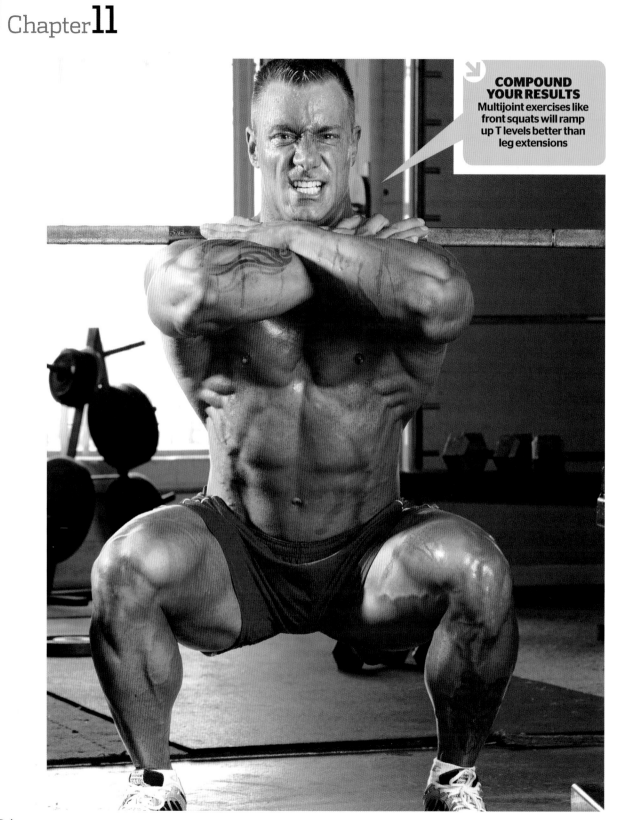

COMPOUND YOUR RESULTS
Multijoint exercises like front squats will ramp up T levels better than leg extensions

→ RULE 2
TRAIN MULTIPLE MUSCLE GROUPS IN EACH WORKOUT

This rationale is based on a study by Danish researchers that found when guys did a biceps-only workout, their testosterone levels didn't budge. When they trained biceps and legs, however, their T levels shot up about 40%.

If the muscle groups are small, such as biceps and triceps, you'll need to add another bodypart to get the testosterone boost. Legs, on the other hand, are such a large group that you could train them alone and still benefit from elevated test levels.

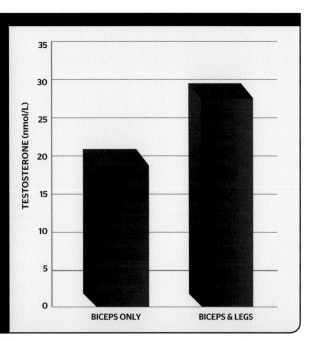

→ RULE 3
WORK MULTIJOINT EXERCISES INTO YOUR WORKOUTS

Using multijoint moves is a simple way to target different muscle groups. This approach keeps you in check with Rule No. 2, and since multijoint exercises allow you to move heavier weight, you'll also be following Rule No. 1.

RAMPED-UP RECEPTORS

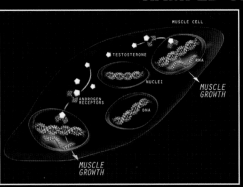

Androgen receptor levels during normal testosterone levels

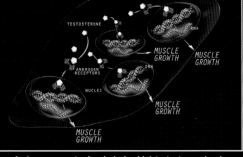

Androgen receptor levels during high testosterone levels

This illustration shows that when testosterone levels shoot up during a test-boosting workout, so does the amount of androgen receptors inside muscle cells. When testosterone docks onto these receptors, it gets a free pass into the nuclei of the muscle cells where it activates genes that increase muscle growth. When testosterone levels and androgen receptor levels are both increased, so is muscle growth.

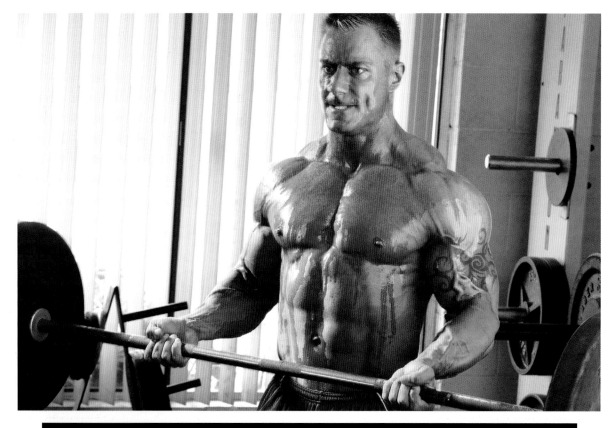

→ RULE 4
PUMP UP THE VOLUME

New Zealand researchers had trained men follow three different squat workouts: 10 sets of 10 reps using 75% 1RM (100 reps total), six sets of four reps using about 90% 1RM (24 reps total), and eight sets of six reps using 45% 1RM (48 reps total).

The scientists found that testosterone levels increased by about 90% in subjects who did the first workout, but saw very little or no change in those doing the other two routines. They suggested that training volume is key in boosting T since neither the 24- nor the 48-rep workout produced much testosterone.

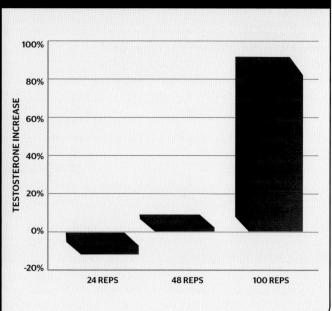

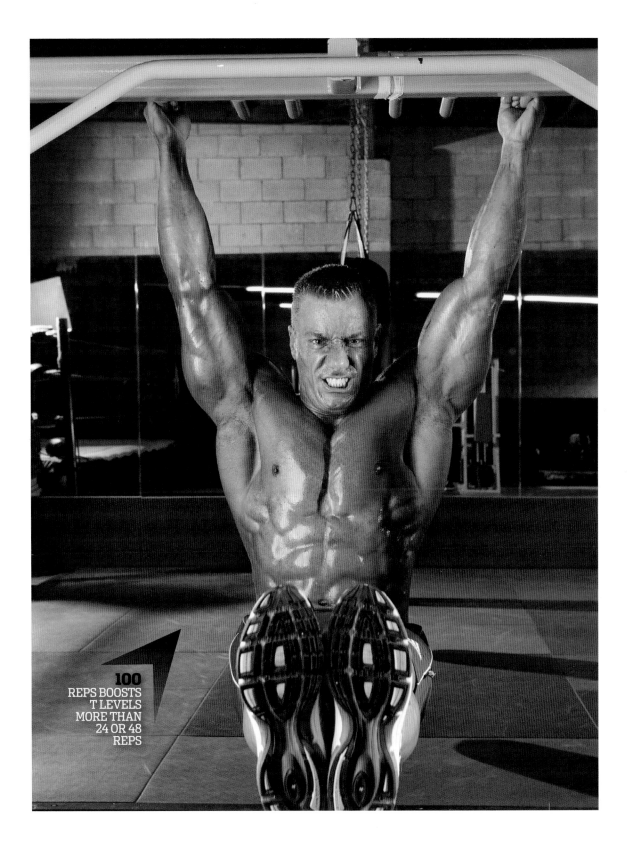

100
REPS BOOSTS
T LEVELS
MORE THAN
24 OR 48
REPS

→ RULE 5
REST LESS

If you sit around yapping with your gym buddies between sets, your test levels may suffer along with your muscle growth. Research shows that testosterone levels rose when subjects rested one minute between sets, but the longer they rested after that, the lower their T sank. Keep rest between sets to about a minute — that should give you enough time to recover so you can train heavy and intensely without compromising your testosterone levels.

GO HEAVY, GO WIDE
Adding weight to your pull-ups will help you add size in your lats and middle back

THE TRAINING FOR MR. T WORKOUT

This workout follows a four-day split so you have ample time to recover, which is another important factor in maximizing testosterone levels. Follow this plan for 4–6 weeks, then change it up using the five golden rules.

WORKOUT 1 MONDAY

EXERCISE	SETS/REPS	REST
Chest		
Dumbbell Bench Press[1]	4/8	1 min.
Smith Machine Decline Press	4/10	1 min.
Cable Crossover	4/12	1 min.
Push-Up	3/to failure	—
— superset with —		
Decline Push-Up	3/to failure	1 min.
Triceps		
Close-Grip Bench Press[1]	4/6	1 min.
Lying Triceps Extension	4/8	1 min.
Pushdown	4/12	1 min.
Dip	2/to failure	1 min.
Abs		
Tri-Set:		
Hanging Leg Raise	4/to failure	—
Hanging Knee Raise	4/to failure	—
Crunch	4/to failure	1 min.

WORKOUT 2 TUESDAY

EXERCISE	SETS/REPS	REST
Back		
Barbell Row[1]	4/6	1 min.
Pull-Up	4/to failure	1 min.
One-Arm Dumbbell Row	4/10	1 min.
Reverse-Grip Lat Pulldown	4/8	1 min.
Seated Cable Row	4/12	1 min.
Biceps		
Barbell Curl[1]	4/6	1 min.
Dumbbell Incline Curl	4/8	1 min.
Cable Curl	4/12	—
— superset with —		
Rope Hammer Curl	4/12	1 min.
Forearms		
Barbell Wrist Curl	4/12	—
— superset with —		
Barbell Reverse Wrist Curl	4/12	1 min.

THE TRAINING FOR MR. T WORKOUT (cont.)

WORKOUT 3 THURSDAY

EXERCISE	SETS/REPS	REST
Shoulders		
Seated Dumbbell Overhead Press[1]	4/6	1 min.
Barbell Overhead Press	4/8	1 min.
Dumbbell Upright Row	4/10	1 min.
Tri-Set:		
Bent-Over Lateral Raise	4/12	—
Lateral Raise	4/12	—
Front Raise	4/12	1 min.
Traps		
Smith Machine Behind-the-Back Shrug	4/10	—
— superset with —		
Smith Machine Shrug	4/10	1 min.
Abs		
Tri-Set:		
Reverse Crunch	4/to failure	—
Crunch	4/to failure	—
Plank	4/60 sec.	1 min.

WORKOUT 4 FRIDAY

EXERCISE	SETS/REPS	REST
Legs		
Squat[1]	4/6	1 min.
Front Squat	4/8	1 min.
Leg Press	4/10	1 min.
Lunge	4/12	1 min.
Romanian Deadlift	4/8	1 min.
Lying Leg Curl	4/15	—
— superset with —		
Leg Extension	4/15	1 min.
Calves		
Standing Calf Raise	4/20	—
— superset with —		
Seated Calf Raise	4/20	1 min.

[1] Do two warm-up sets using a weight with which you can complete 20–30 reps. Perform 5–8 reps as fast and explosively as possible on the positive portion, and slow and controlled on the negative portion.

← SMITH MACHINE BEHIND-THE-BACK SHRUG

Stand in a Smith machine with your feet shoulder-width apart. Set the bar just under your glutes and grasp it behind you. Keeping your chest up and abs tight, unlock the bar and shrug your shoulders straight up, squeezing your traps at the top. Slowly reverse the motion to return to the start.

Chapter 12

Upper-Body Blast

Developing a titanic torso doesn't have to take forever. This month-long plan will help you pack on serious pounds, and add inches to your chest and back in no time

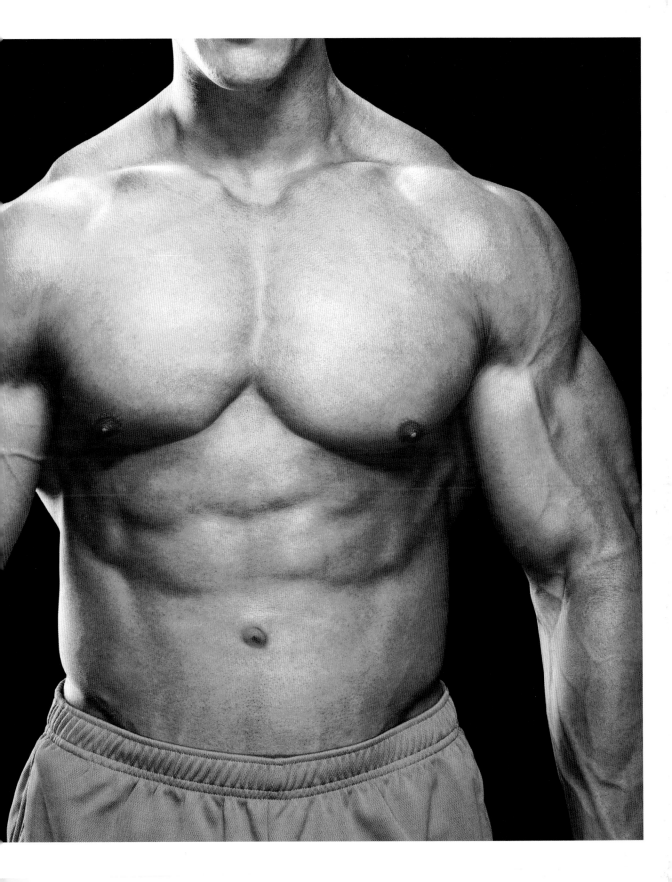

IF YOUR GOAL IS TO LEAVE A LASTING impression — whether you're coming or going — you need a king-size chest and a larger-than-life back.

Packing on the right amount of muscle from front to back means using the best mass-building exercises and a mix of rep ranges so you leave no stone — or in this case muscle fiber — unturned. "The general school of thought is that muscle growth occurs by doing moderate amounts of reps," says C.J. Murphy, MFS, CISSN, national powerlifting champion and owner of Total Performance Sports (Everett, Massachusetts). "The truth is, if you want your chest and back to get big, you need to do enough moderate-rep work to stimulate growth along with enough low-rep, heavy-load work to increase your strength." This workout does just that and much more.

TORSO TRIFECTA

One advantage of Murphy's routine is that it targets the chest and back twice a week, and every other bodypart once. "If you want to build up a specific muscle group, you need to hit it hard with the right volume, then back off and give it plenty of rest," Murphy says. He believes most guys do too much, which can limit their ability to grow. By punishing your chest and back only twice weekly — and limiting how often you train other bodyparts — you'll give them all the time they need to recharge and get large.

The order of exercises is also important. You'll train heavy with barbells and dumbbells on one day, and do bodyweight/isolation movements for higher reps on the other. "Many lifters never bother training their slow-twitch muscle fibers using higher-rep, lighter-weight moves because they know the fast-twitch fibers are capable of growing more effectively," Murphy says.

> ## If you want to earn stares, you have to earn inches

"Since slow-twitch fibers can still grow 15%–20%, targeting both consistently can maximize your growth potential."

Finally, there are a significant number of bodyweight movements (dips, inverted rows, pull-ups, push-ups) in the routine. "Using these exercises on a regular basis teaches your muscles to work together," Murphy says. "The more in sync they are, the more effectively they'll assist each other on heavy free-weight days, so you can push, pull or press even more."

MAKING EVERY SET COUNT

"To grow big, you need to go heavy, but many trainees never reach their potential because they warm up the wrong way," says Murphy, who insists that warm-up sets should never be volume-oriented. "Treating warm-up sets like working sets only robs your muscles of strength they could use during your workout. Instead, do only enough reps to get your body accustomed to the movement."

First warm up for 5–10 minutes with a cardio activity of your choice. Then, on any exercise that requires heavy sets of 3–8 reps, follow this protocol: Use just the bar (or a weight that's 10%–15% of your one-rep max, 1RM, for dumbbells) and do 5–10 reps; increase the weight to 30%–35% of your 1RM and do three reps; go up to 45%–50% of your 1RM and do three reps; and finally, use a weight that's 70%–75% of your 1RM and do one rep. For example, if you're a 300-pound bencher, start with an empty bar and do 5–10 reps; add a 25-pound plate to each side (95 pounds) for three reps; load the bar with 145 pounds and do three reps; increase that to 225 pounds and do one rep; then start your working sets.

"Instead of feeling fried at the end of each warm-up, your muscles will be fresh," Murphy points out. "You'll instantly handle more weight than usual with proper form — the perfect game plan for overloading your muscles so they get strong fast and grow big even faster."

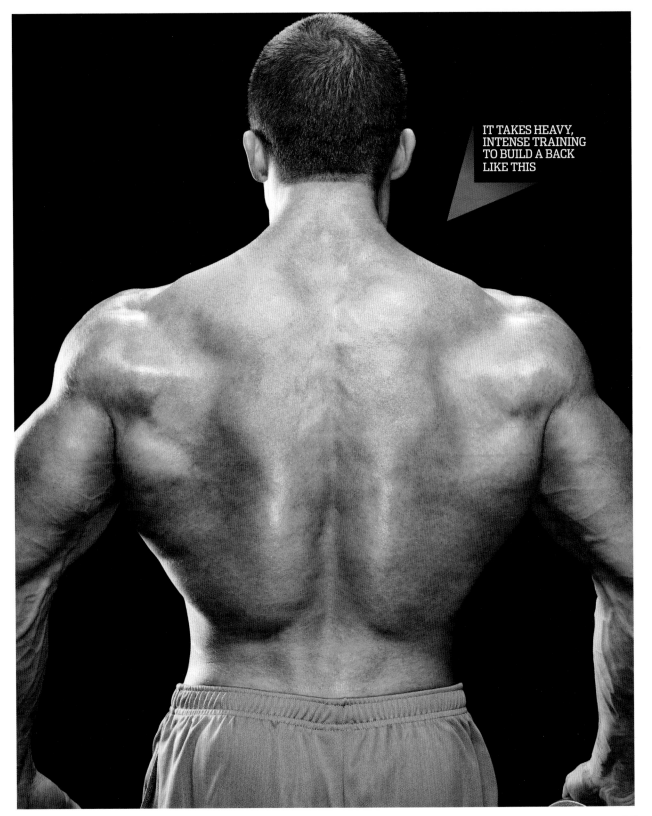

IT TAKES HEAVY,
INTENSE TRAINING
TO BUILD A BACK
LIKE THIS

INVERTED ROW →

Start: Place a flat bench sideways a few feet in front of a Smith machine and set the bar to about waist level. Grasp the bar with a shoulder-width grip, place your heels on the bench and let yourself hang from the bar, arms extended. Your body should form a straight line from head to heels.

Execution: With your elbows in, slowly pull your chest up to the bar. Hold for a second, then slowly lower yourself to full-arm extension. Keep your body rigid throughout.

TIP
Pull your navel toward your spine and squeeze your glutes to help stabilize your body

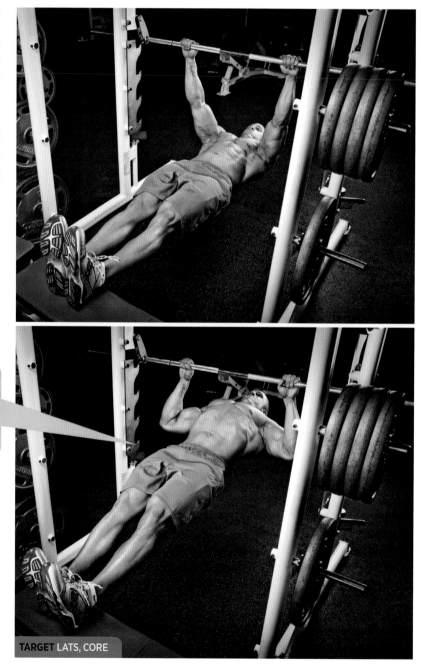

TARGET LATS, CORE

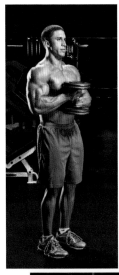

← CHEST-LOADED LUNGE

Start: Stand erect with your feet hip-width apart and hold a heavy dumbbell in front of your chest, with your elbows out to your sides.
Execution: Step forward with your left foot, then descend until your left thigh is parallel to the floor. Drive through your left heel to return to standing. Bring your feet together, then step forward with your right foot.

TIP
Keep your chest up as you descend. Don't allow the weight to pull your torso forward

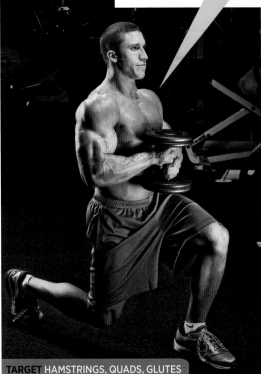

TARGET HAMSTRINGS, QUADS, GLUTES

MONTH-LONG PLAN WEEK 1

DAY	EXERCISE	SETS	REPS/DISTANCE
1	Barbell Deadlift	3	7–8,5–6,3–4[1]
	Barbell Row	3	7–8,5–6,3–4[1]
	Heavy Shrug	3	7–8,5–6,3–4[1]
	Weighted Dip	3	7–8,5–6,3–4[1,2]
	Push-Up	1	75[3]
	Cable Crossover	2	12–15
	Svend Press	2	12–15
2	**Off**		
3	Barbell Squat	3	7–8,5–6,3–4[1]
	Keystone Deadlift	3	7–8,5–6,3–4[1]
	Chest-Loaded Lunge	3	7–8,5–6,3–4[1]
	Weighted Back Extension	2	8–12
4	**Off**		
5	Heavy Barbell Incline Press	3	7–8,5–6,3–4[1]
	Dumbbell Decline Press	3	7–8,5–6,3–4[1]
	Overhead Press	3	10–12
	Weighted Pull-Up	3	7–8,5–6,3–4[1,2]
	Inverted Row	1	60[3]
	Face Pull	2	12–15
	Standing Low-Cable Rope Row	2	12–15
6	**Walking Overhead Press**	**3**	**50 ft.**
	Lateral Raise	3	10,10–12,12–15[4]
	Tate Press	3	8–10
	— superset with —		
	Pushdown	3	12–15
	Low-Cable Towel Curl	3	8–10
	— superset with —		
	Standing Hammer Curl	3	12–15
	Donkey Calf Raise	3	12–15,8–10,6–8[1]
7	**Off**		

[1] Do pyramid-style, increasing the weight after each set.
[2] Immediately after your last set, drop the weight and rep to failure using only your bodyweight.
[3] Do as many reps as you can as quickly as possible, stopping just short of failure; rest as many seconds as the number of reps you have left, then continue.
[4] Perform as drop sets: On each set, do as many reps as you can with your heaviest weight, then decrease the weight as needed to get the prescribed number of reps.

MONTH-LONG PLAN WEEK 2

DAY	EXERCISE	SETS	REPS/DISTANCE
1	Barbell Deadlift	3	7–8,5–6,3–4[1]
	Barbell Row	3	7–8,5–6,3–4[1]
	Heavy Shrug	3	7–8,5–6,3–4[1]
	Weighted Dip	4	7–8,5–6,3–4[1,2]
	Push-Up	1	100[3]
	Cable Crossover	3	12–15
	Svend Press	3	12–15
2	**Off**		
3	Barbell Squat	3	7–8,5–6,3–4[1]
	Keystone Deadlift	3	7–8,5–6,3–4[1]
	Chest-Loaded Lunge	3	7–8,5–6,3–4[1]
	Weighted Back Exten.	3	8–12
4	**Off**		
5	Heavy Barbell Incline Press	3	7–8,5–6,3–4[1]
	Dumbbell Decline Press	3	7–8,5–6,3–4[1]
	Overhead Press	3	10–12
	Weighted Pull-Up	4	7–8,5–6,3–4[1,2]
	Inverted Row	1	85[3]
	Face Pull	3	12–15
	Standing Low-Cable Rope Row	3	12–15
6	Walking Overhead Press	3	60 ft.
	Lateral Raise	3	10,10–12,12–15[4]
	Tate Press	4	8–10
	— superset with —		
	Pushdown	4	12–15
	Low-Cable Towel Curl	4	8–10
	— superset with —		
	Standing Hammer Curl	4	12–15
	Donkey Calf Raise	3	12–15,8–10,6–8[1]
7	**Off**		

[1] Do pyramid-style, increasing the weight after each set.
[2] Immediately after your last set, drop the weight and rep to failure using only your bodyweight.
[3] Do as many reps as you can as quickly as possible, stopping just short of failure; rest as many seconds as the number of reps you have left, then continue.
[4] Perform as drop sets: On each set, do as many reps as you can with your heaviest weight, then decrease the weight as needed to get the prescribed number of reps.

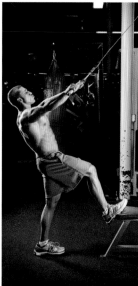

← FACE PULL

Start: Stand in front of a lat pulldown station and grasp the long bar with an overhand grip, hands wider than shoulder width. Place one foot on the seat and lean back so your body is at a 45-degree angle.
Execution: Squeeze your shoulder blades together, then slowly pull the bar toward your face. Hold the contraction, then slowly resist the bar's return to the start position.

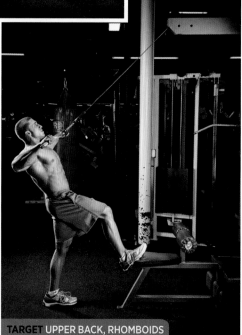

TARGET UPPER BACK, RHOMBOIDS

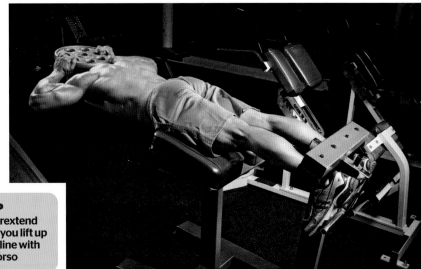

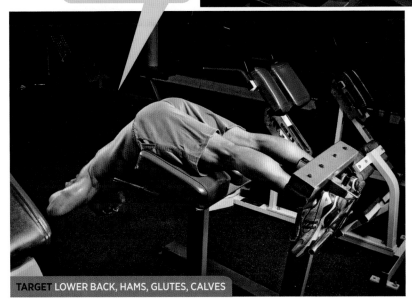

TIP
Don't hyperextend your neck as you lift up — keep it in line with your torso

← WEIGHTED BACK EXTENSION

Start: Lie facedown on a hyperextension bench with your thighs on the pads and your ankles secured under the footpads. Your body should form a straight line from head to heels. Hold a weight plate behind your head.

Execution: Keeping your back flat, bend at the hips until your torso is perpendicular to the floor, then contract your hams and glutes to return to the start.

TARGET LOWER BACK, HAMS, GLUTES, CALVES

MONTH-LONG PLAN WEEK 3

DAY	EXERCISE	SETS	REPS/DISTANCE
1	Barbell Deadlift	3	7-8,5-6,3-4[1]
	Barbell Row	3	7-8,5-6,3-4[1]
	Heavy Shrug	3	7-8,5-6,3-4[1]
	Weighted Dip	5	7-8,6-7,5-6,4-5,3-4[1,2]
	Push-Up	1	125[3]
	Cable Crossover	4	12-15
	Svend Press	4	12-15
2	**Off**		
3	Barbell Squat	4	7-8,5-6,4-5,3-4[1]
	Keystone Deadlift	4	7-8,5-6,4-5,3-4[1]
	Chest-Loaded Lunge	4	7-8,5-6,4-5,3-4[1]
	Weighted Back Exten.	4	8-12
4	**Off**		
5	Heavy Barbell Incline Press	3	7-8,5-6,3-4[1]
	Dumbbell Decline Press	3	7-8,5-6,3-4[1]
	Overhead Press	3	10-12
	Weighted Pull-Up	5	7-8,6-7,5-6,4-5,3-4[1,2]
	Inverted Row	1	110[3]
	Face Pull	4	12-15
	Standing Low-Cable Rope Row	4	12-15
6	**Walking Overhead Press**	3	70 ft.
	Lateral Raise	3	10,10-12,12-15[4]
	Tate Press — superset with —	5	8-10
	Pushdown	5	12-15
	Low-Cable Towel Curl — superset with —	5	8-10
	Standing Hammer Curl	5	12-15
	Donkey Calf Raise	3	12-15,8-10,6-8[1]
7	**Off**		

[1] Do pyramid-style, increasing the weight after each set.
[2] Immediately after your last set, drop the weight and rep to failure using only your bodyweight.
[3] Do as many reps as you can as quickly as possible, stopping just short of failure; rest as many seconds as the number of reps you have left, then continue.
[4] Perform as drop sets: On each set, do as many reps as you can with your heaviest weight, then decrease the weight as needed to get the prescribed number of reps.

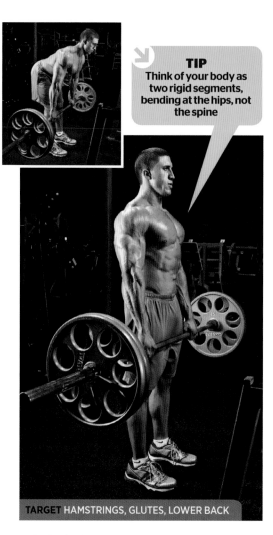

> **TIP**
> Think of your body as two rigid segments, bending at the hips, not the spine

TARGET HAMSTRINGS, GLUTES, LOWER BACK

↑ KEYSTONE DEADLIFT

Start: Set the barbell in a power rack to about mid-thigh level. Grasp the bar with an overhand, shoulder-width grip, take two steps back and hold it in front of your thighs. Stand erect with your feet about hip-width apart and knees slightly bent.
Execution: With your lower back arched slightly, bend at the hips and push your glutes back, keeping the bar in contact with your legs. Stop when the bar reaches your knees, pause, then drive through your heels and push your hips forward to return to the start.

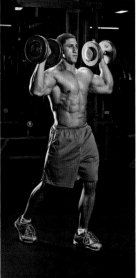

← WALKING OVERHEAD PRESS

Start: Stand erect holding a dumbbell in each hand in front of your shoulders, palms forward.
Execution: Walk forward and press the weights overhead, then lower them back to your shoulders. Don't worry about synching your steps and presses; just press the dumbbells as many times as you can in the prescribed number of steps.

MONTH-LONG PLAN WEEK 4

DAY	EXERCISE	SETS	REPS/DISTANCE
1	Barbell Deadlift	3	7–8,5–6,3–4[1]
	Barbell Row	3	7–8,5–6,3–4[1]
	Heavy Shrug	3	7–8,5–6,3–4[1]
	Weighted Dip	5	7–8,6–7,5–6,4–5,3–4[1,2]
	Push-Up	1	125[3]
	Cable Crossover	5	12–15
	Svend Press	5	12–15
2	Off		
3	Barbell Squat	4	7–8,5–6,4–5,3–4[1]
	Keystone Deadlift	4	7–8,5–6,4–5,3–4[1]
	Chest-Loaded Lunge	4	7–8,5–6,4–5,3–4[1]
	Weighted Back Exten.	5	8–12
4	Off		
5	Heavy Barbell Incline Press	3	7–8,5–6,3–4[1]
	Dumbbell Decline Press	3	7–8,5–6,3–4[1]
	Overhead Press	3	10–12
	Weighted Pull-Up	5	7–8,6–7,5–6,4–5,3–4[1,2]
	Inverted Row	1	135[3]
	Face Pull	5	12–15
	Standing Low-Cable Rope Row	5	12–15
6	Walking Overhead Press	3	80 ft.
	Lateral Raise	3	10,10–12,12–15[4]
	Tate Press	5	8–10
	— superset with —		
	Pushdown	5	12–15
	Low-Cable Towel Curl	5	8–10
	— superset with —		
	Standing Hammer Curl	5	12–15
	Donkey Calf Raise	3	12–15,8–10,6–8[1]
7	Off		

[1] Do pyramid-style, increasing the weight after each set.
[2] Immediately after your last set, drop the weight and rep to failure using only your bodyweight.
[3] Do as many reps as you can as quickly as possible, stopping just short of failure; rest as many seconds as the number of reps you have left, then continue.
[4] Perform as drop sets: On each set, do as many reps as you can with your heaviest weight, then decrease the weight as needed to get the prescribed number of reps.

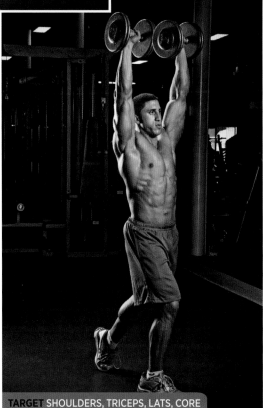

TARGET SHOULDERS, TRICEPS, LATS, CORE

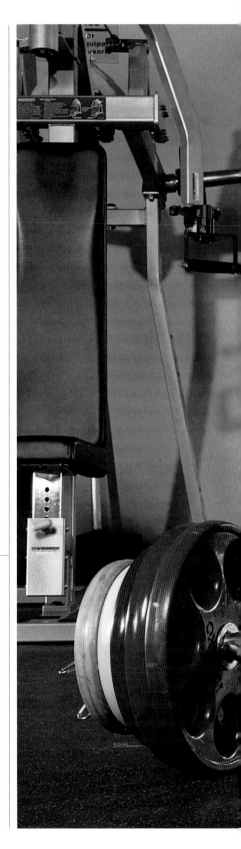

Chapter 13

Get a Leg Up

Grow your lower body from every angle with this triphasic strategy for strength and mass gains

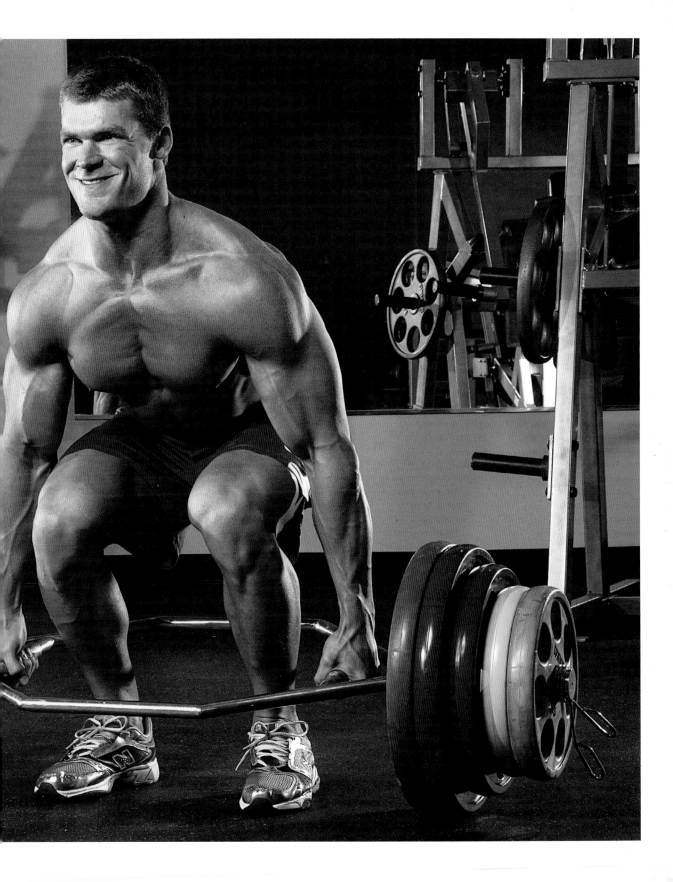

> ## You want to get bigger? Wake up and realize that you must get stronger first.

STRONG WORDS FROM TEAM STALEY

(Gilbert, Arizona) coach and powerlifter Phil Stevens, who has deadlifted 700-plus pounds in competition at a bodyweight of 275 pounds. It's with this in mind that triphasic training was developed — three phases in a six-week program, each designed to ensure that you get progressively bigger and stronger.

In the first phase — the priming phase — you build your body with basic lifts, working up to very heavy weights and low reps. You should progress by 5% per week, which doesn't sound like much but is actually significant for most people. "There's no better way to grow, from head to toe, than putting heavy loads on your body," Stevens notes.

The reps are performed quickly, with long rest periods between sets to ensure optimal recovery, so you can hit the target muscles just as hard in the next set. One exception is the overhead squat, which is part warm-up and part preparation for the heavier loads you'll use in subsequent weeks. Only after you master the form can you truly reap its benefits.

Phase 2 is a necessary deload phase, where you decrease weight and volume to give your body a break and prepare it for what's to come. "A short and effective deload resets both body and mind, allowing you to fully realize the progress you've made in the preceding weeks," Stevens explains.

Exercises in this phase are performed with light weight at a rhythmic pace. Limit rest periods to less than two minutes, just enough to get the blood flowing. Including unilateral moves takes advantage of the physiological phenomenon known as the bilateral deficit, which means you get a better muscle contraction when using just one arm or leg than you would with both. This increases your muscle-fiber recruitment without too much effort.

Fresh off the deload week, the shock phase is where you'll really progress. "I relate the shock phase to a competition," Stevens says. "It's what those previous weeks of hard work and recovery have prepped you for."

Sets are very heavy to maximally stress the muscles and drive your growth as much as possible. Every aspect of your strength will be worked in these two weeks; they'll be taxing, but you'll be ready. Maintain at least a 5% progression between weeks and you'll see the difference.

TRIPHASIC TRAINING PROGRAM

PRIMING PHASE — WEEKS 1-3

EXERCISE	SETS	REPS	LOAD
Overhead Squat (warm-up)	2	8	Broomstick
Front Squat	5	3	6RM
Deadlift	5	3	6RM
Dumbbell Snatch	3 per arm	3	8RM
Pillar-Assisted Manual Leg Curl	2	6	Bodyweight

DELOAD PHASE — WEEK 4

EXERCISE	SETS	REPS	LOAD
Overhead Squat (warm-up)	2	6	up to 45 lbs.
High Pull	2	6	15RM
Bulgarian Squat	2 per leg	8	20 RM
One-Leg Romanian Deadlift	2 per leg	8	20RM
One-Leg Curl	2 per leg	10	20RM

SHOCK PHASE — WEEKS 5-6

EXERCISE	SETS	REPS	LOAD
Overhead Squat (warm-up)	3	3	6RM
Trap-Bar Deadlift & Farmer's Walk	5	5	6RM
Hip Lift	3 per leg	8	Bodyweight
Dumbbell Thruster	3	8	12RM
Band-Assisted Manual Leg Curl	3	6	Bodyweight

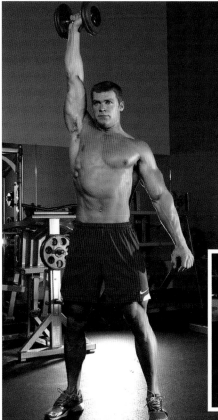

← DUMBBELL SNATCH

Start: With your feet shoulder-width apart and a dumbbell between them, squat down to grasp the weight in one hand.
Execution: Begin the pull much like you would in a deadlift, gradually accelerating the dumbbell as it approaches your knees. Once the weight's at knee level, extend your body, shrug and thrust it overhead as if to throw it through the ceiling. Repeat for reps, then switch sides.

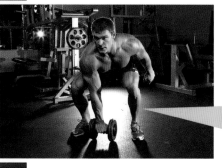

TIP
The snatch is an explosive move, never to be done slowly. Your arm stays straight and the weight travels overhead in one fluid motion

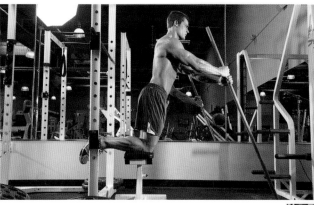

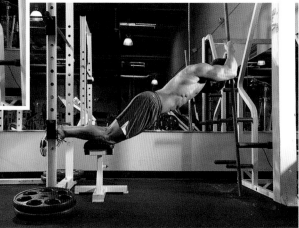

PILLAR-ASSISTED MANUAL LEG CURL →

Start: Stand one end of an empty barbell or broomstick on the floor. Kneel facing it either with a bar anchored over your Achilles or backward at a lat pulldown station with your feet under the rollers. **Execution:** Keeping your body straight from knees to head, lower your torso toward the floor until it's nearly parallel. Contract your hamstrings and use the pillar for support to return to the start position.

Chapter 13

HIGH PULL →

Start: Stand erect with your feet hip-width apart. Squat down and grasp a barbell in front of your shins with your arms extended and hands shoulder-width apart.

Execution: In one explosive motion, extend your knees and hips as you pull the bar as high as possible, leading with your elbows as in an upright row. Let the weight drop back to the start position, settle yourself, then begin the next rep. Set a moderate height mark and lift the bar to it every time.

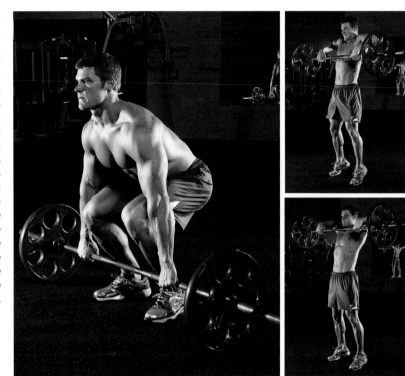

← BULGARIAN SQUAT

Start: Stand erect holding a light dumbbell in each hand, and place the toes or top of one foot on a bench behind you. Most of your weight should be on your front leg.

Execution: Bend your front knee and squat until your thigh is slightly past parallel to the floor. If your shin isn't perpendicular to the floor at the bottom, step forward. Drive up through your front heel to return to standing, using your back leg only as support. Repeat for reps, then switch legs.

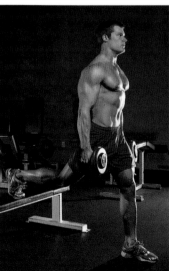

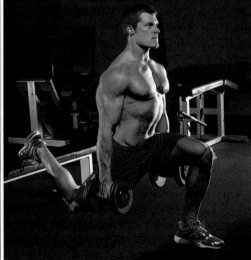

ONE-LEG ROMANIAN DEADLIFT →

Start: Stand erect holding a dumbbell in each hand with your weight on one leg.

Execution: Keeping your chest up, abs tight and the natural arch in your low back, drive your hips back and lift your nonworking leg behind you to lower your torso until it's roughly parallel to the floor. Your leg and torso should be in line. Keeping your back flat and head neutral, contract your hamstring and glute, and lift your torso while pushing your hips forward to return to standing. Let your back leg lower to the floor without touching down. Repeat for reps, then switch sides. For a greater challenge, lift your knee at the end of each rep.

TIP
Focusing on a point on the floor with your eyes will help you maintain balance as you lower down and raise up in a controlled fashion

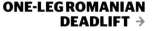

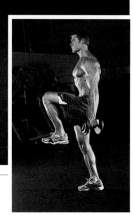

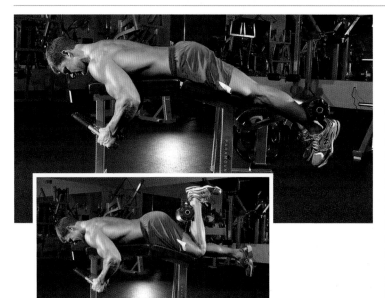

← ONE-LEG CURL

Start: Lie facedown on a leg-curl machine and position your Achilles below the roller, your knees just off the edge of the bench. Keep them slightly bent here to prevent overextension.

Execution: Grasp the sides of the bench or handles for stability. Contract your hamstring to raise your foot toward your glute in a strong, deliberate motion. Squeeze at the top, then return to the start. Repeat for reps, then switch sides.

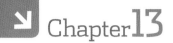

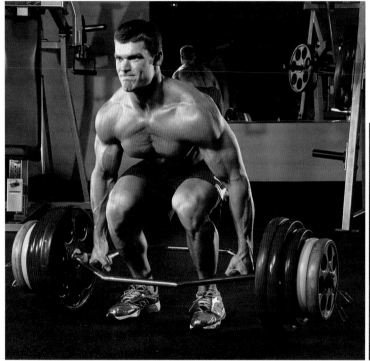

← TRAP-BAR DEADLIFT & FARMER'S WALK

Perform a conventional deadlift with a trap bar for reps, then take 10 steps with the weight. Use heavy dumbbells if you don't have access to a trap bar.

BAND-ASSISTED MANUAL LEG CURL →

Start: Anchor a band around a stable object at chest level, and wrap the loop under your armpits. Kneel on a bench or the floor with your feet anchored. **Execution:** Hold the band in place with your thumbs and lower your torso toward the floor until it's nearly parallel, keeping your body straight from knees to head. Squeeze your hamstrings to return to the start. For optimal safety, have a bench in front of you at the fully extended position.

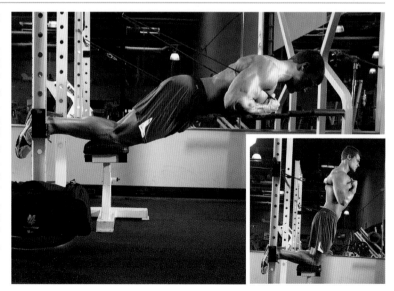

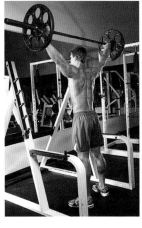

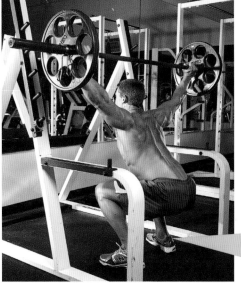

← OVERHEAD SQUAT

Start: Stand erect with your feet shoulder-width apart. Grasp a barbell using a wide, overhand grip and lift it overhead.
Execution: With your elbows locked and the bar slightly behind your head, bend your knees and hips to descend as in a traditional squat, keeping your back flat and your knees tracking forward. Drive through your heels to return to the start.

TIP
Because of the advanced nature of this exercise, start off very light if you've never done overhead squats before

HIP LIFT (NOT PICTURED)

Start: Lie faceup with your upper back perpendicular on a bench and your feet flat on the floor.
Execution: Raise one leg, keeping your knee bent, until your thigh is perpendicular to the floor. With your hips below shoulder level, contract your glutes and hamstrings to lift your hips to shoulder level or higher. Repeat for reps, then switch sides.

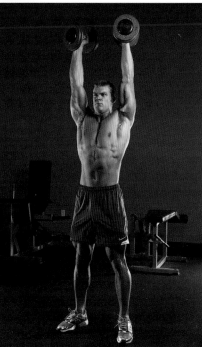

DUMBBELL THRUSTER →

Start: Hold a pair of dumbbells in overhead-press position, with your wrists flexed.
Execution: Descend into a traditional front squat, then on the ascent use your momentum to simultaneously press the weights overhead.

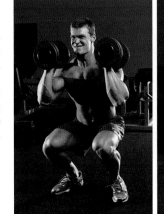

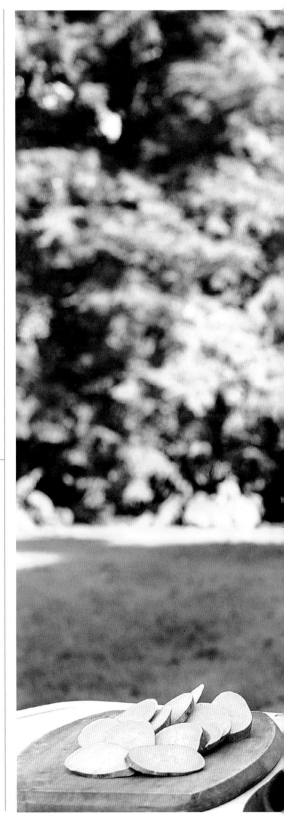

Chapter 14

Eat Big

Make sure the food you eat turns into rock-hard muscle with these 18 guidelines

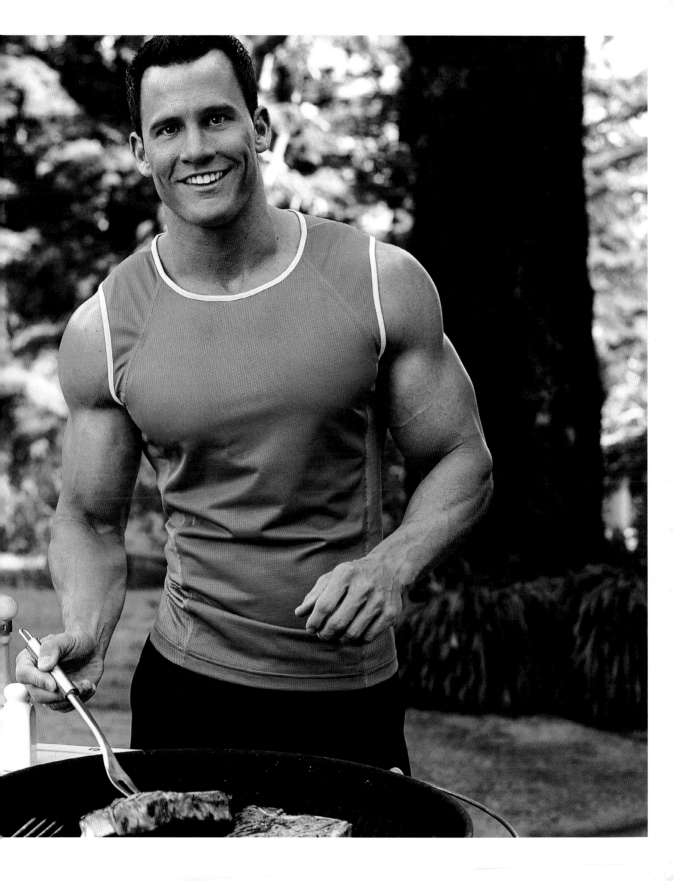

HERE'S SOME SIMPLE MATH THAT MANY PEOPLE STILL CAN'T SEEM TO GRASP.
You're in the gym for only an hour or so each day, leaving another 22–23 hours in which muscle growth depends solely on what goes in — or stays out of — your piehole. So why is the nutrition side of the mass-gaining equation often marginalized? It's probably because the bench press is a lot sexier than a spinach salad. But if you want to take your physique from string bean to Mr. Clean, certain dietary guidelines need your utmost attention. These 18 get-big eating tips will help you build the body you've always yearned for without blowing up like the Pillsbury Doughboy.

PACK IN PROTEIN
Protein provides the amino acids used as building blocks for muscle growth. To keep it going full force, shoot for 1-1.5 grams of protein per pound of bodyweight, or 180-270 grams a day for the 180-pounder. Top protein picks include dairy, eggs, poultry, red meat and seafood, not to mention whey, casein and soy protein powders. These foods offer a wealth of complete protein, providing your muscles with the essential aminos necessary for recovery and growth.

RISE & DINE
When trying to gain mass, eat two breakfasts. To restock liver glycogen and put the brakes on catabolism that chips away at your muscle overnight, down two scoops of whey protein along with a fast-digesting carb such as sugar, Vitargo or white bread immediately upon waking. One of our favorite morning shakes is 2 cups of coffee, 2 scoops of whey and 2–3 tablespoons of sugar. About 60 minutes later, follow up with a whole-food breakfast that boasts quality protein such as Canadian bacon or eggs and slower-burning carbs such as oatmeal or whole-grain toast to provide sustained energy.

MUNCH BEFORE BED
Before hitting the sack, eat a snack of slow-digesting casein protein and healthy fat. Casein coagulates in the gut, ensuring a steady supply of amino acids to your muscles to slow catabolism as you sleep. Some fat will further slow digestion. About 30 minutes before bedtime, have 20–40 grams of casein protein powder or 1 cup of low-fat cottage cheese (a stellar casein source) mixed with 2 tablespoons flaxseed oil, or 1–2 ounces of nuts or seeds. Avoid late-night carbs; they can mess with overnight growth-hormone release and promote fat gain.

EAT REAL FOOD

To quote America's foremost food writer Michael Pollan, "Don't eat anything your grandmother wouldn't recognize as food." Protein powders notwithstanding, this is great advice. In general, whole foods including lean meats, nuts and vegetables contain more nutrients muscles crave, and deliver a steadier supply of amino acids and blood glucose to muscles than the nutritional dreck found in the middle aisles of your local supermarket.

PLAN AHEAD

Coming home ravenous after a balls-out training session and having nothing prepared can send you on a hunt for the nearest bag of Doritos. But having a stockpile of protein-packed foods that can be reheated easily ensures you make healthy choices and get the nutrients your muscles need. Use the weekend to rustle up big batches of chicken, chili, hard-boiled eggs and pasta, which will keep in the fridge or freezer during the week ahead. Also, write down your week's menu in advance so you can get everything you need from the market or grocer in one shot.

WEIGH IN

Forget eyeballing portions. To be precise about your calorie and protein intakes, add a digital food scale to your arsenal of kitchen tools (try the EatSmart Nutrition Scale; $75, eatsmartproducts.com). This is the most accurate way to determine the proper serving sizes of foods such as cheeses and meats. For instance, you don't want your chicken breast to be a measly 3 ounces, but you also don't want to plop an elephantine 12-ounce steak on your plate.

FACE THE FATS

Fat, including much-maligned saturated fat, is necessary for building a rock-solid physique: It revs up testosterone production and helps your joints endure the heavy lifting needed to spur muscle expansion. Aim for at least 0.5 gram of fat per pound of bodyweight (90 grams for a 180-pound man) or 30% of total daily calories. Divide that into equal thirds coming from the primary T-booster sat fats found in beef, coconut products and dairy; monounsaturated fats from almonds, avocado, olive oil and peanut butter; and fat-burning polyunsaturated fats found in fatty fish, flaxseeds, hempseeds and walnuts. Avoid the trans-fatty acids in many fried and commercially packaged foods.

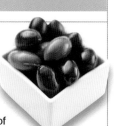

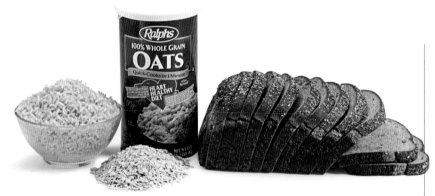

DON'T SHUN CARBS

Muscle can't live on protein alone. To gain mass, you must eat plenty of carbohydrates: 2–3 grams per pound of bodyweight per day. Carbs contain the calories required for growth, and glycogen to fuel intense lifting and keep muscles looking full. Good slow-digesting options for most meals are brown rice, oatmeal, quinoa, sprouted bread, sweet potatoes and whole-grain pasta to keep insulin and energy levels steady. The exception to this rule is your first meal of the day and postworkout snack when you want fast-digesting carbs such as fruit, fruit juice, refined bread and pasta, white potatoes and white rice. That's when an insulin spike is desirable to channel amino acids and other nutrients into muscles, setting the table for anabolism and recovery.

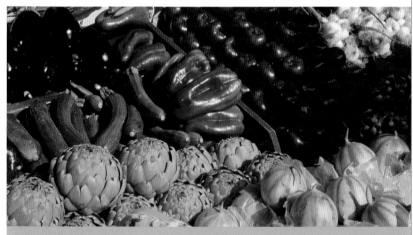

HIT THE FARM

Not just for "granola" types, farmers' markets are often the best places to find muscle-building whole foods such as eggs, meats and vegetables that haven't been treated with hormones or pesticides. Prices also tend to be cheaper when you buy direct from the farmer, meaning you won't have to skimp on staples. Luckily, farmers' markets are springing up like dandelions on a pesticide-free lawn. Go to localharvest.org to find one in your neck of the woods.

EAT WHEY PROTEIN PRE- & POSTWORKOUT

In a study published in the journal *Amino Acids*, Finnish scientists discovered that weightlifters who consumed whey protein before and immediately after workouts produced more of a compound called cyclin-dependent kinase 2, or CDK2, than those who didn't take whey. CDK2 is believed to activate muscle stem cells involved in hypertrophy and recovery from intense training. In addition, a 2009 study by Japanese researchers found that consuming whey and glucose prompted larger stores of post-training muscle glycogen than when subjects ingested just glucose. Shoot for 20–30 grams of fast-digesting whey protein isolate or hydrolysate 30 minutes preworkout and immediately postworkout. Studies suggest that adding 10–20 grams of casein protein to your pre- and postworkout whey shakes can further enhance the anabolic effect.

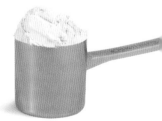

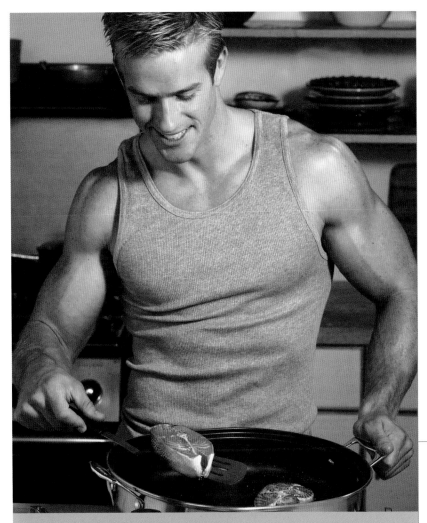

WOLF DOWN ENOUGH CALORIES

You have to eat big to get big. Muscle, unlike flab, is a very metabolically active tissue, and you need to put away plenty of calories to keep it alive and growing. Nibble too few calories and you'll whittle away muscle. When mass gain is the goal, aim to consume about 20 calories per pound of bodyweight each day (about 3,600 calories for a 180-pound guy). Keep an eye on your physique: If you find 20 calories packs on mass and fat, drop to 16–18 calories per pound.

EMBRACE YOUR INNER EMERIL

To retain control over what and how much goes down your gullet, you must prepare the majority of your own meals. Fast food and diner food contain too many menaces to muscle to make them a viable part of a mass-gain diet plan. If the only thing you know how to do in the kitchen is pop open a cold one, seek out a cooking class — or a girlfriend.

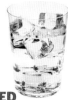

STAY HYDRATED

A critical component of your mass-gaining diet, water helps maintain muscle fullness. After all, muscles contain more H_2O than most other tissues. So follow the National Academy of Sciences, Institute of Medicine's recommendation that men guzzle at least 16 cups of water per day (128 ounces or 1 gallon). It seems like a lot, but it includes the water in fruits, vegetables, milk, soup and fat-burning green tea.

TRACK YOUR INTAKE

The only way you'll know if you're eating enough in the right proportions to grow muscle is to keep a detailed food diary, and tally your calories and macronutrients. The huge database of foods at nutritiondata.com can help you crunch the numbers.

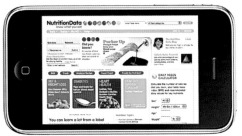

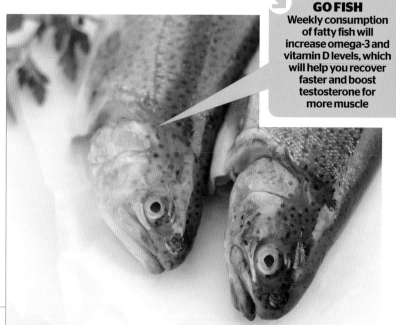

↘
GO FISH
Weekly consumption of fatty fish will increase omega-3 and vitamin D levels, which will help you recover faster and boost testosterone for more muscle

SCHEDULE FREQUENT NOSHING

Eating often will keep you satiated and give your muscles the constant stream of nutrients they need to grow. Not only are hunger pangs a sign that your body may have entered a catabolic state, but when you're starving you're more likely to OD on leftover birthday cake at the office. Try to consume eight physique-friendly meals or snacks throughout the day, including your pre- and postworkout repasts.

GET COLORFUL

A diet should never be monochromatic. It's vital that you eat multicolored fruits and vegetables to ingest a range of antioxidants — the pigments that give produce its bright hues — which aid in muscle recovery and promote growth. A Colorado State University (Fort Collins) study reported that consuming a variety of fruits and veggies containing various phytochemical antioxidants more effectively prevented cell DNA damage, which can slow hypertrophy and initiate disease, than a diet of limited produce. Blueberries, broccoli, carrots, cherries, kale, kiwi and red bell peppers are among the most antioxidant-rich finds in the produce section.

REEL IN FATTY FISH

Show your muscles some love by slicing into fatty fish such as arctic char, mackerel, rainbow trout, salmon and sardines 3-4 times per week. For starters, these swimmers are a good whole-food option postworkout because their protein digests faster than beef, pork and poultry. And since they contain omega-3 fats that help reduce inflammation, these catches of the day could get you back in the squat rack sooner after a killer workout. Plus, Australian researchers discovered that men with the highest blood omega-3 levels had better muscle-to-fat body compositions than those with lower omega-3 levels. Fatty fish are also the best food source of vitamin D. Muscle cells have receptors for the sunshine vitamin and when vitamin D docks at them, it improves muscle function and strength. What's more, low D levels are associated with lower levels of testosterone and higher levels of circulating parathyroid hormone, which encourages fat gain.

GET YOUR GAME ON

Before the mass exodus to cookie-cutter suburbia, game meat was a big part of the American dinner. Sadly, the move to industrial cattle-raising was our loss. Game meats such as bison, elk, ostrich and venison are among the best muscle-building foods around. Besides having a superior protein-to-fat ratio that helps pack on lean mass, most game animals are grass-fed with plenty of room to roam. This produces more fat-burning omega-3s and conjugated linoleic acid. Look for them at farmers' markets or order at eatwild.com.

MUSCLE-BUILDING MEAL PLANS

TRYING TO PACK ON MUSCLE? HERE'S HOW TO LOAD UP YOUR PLATE THROUGHOUT THE DAY WITH GREAT MASS-BUILDING FOODS

When you want to add size, you should take in a hefty number of calories (about 20 per pound of bodyweight per day) that includes 1–1.5 grams of protein per pound. Carbs, which are necessary for recovery and to fuel intense workouts, should come in around 2 grams per pound on training days. Eat at least 0.5 gram of fat per pound, emphasizing healthy fats such as olive oil and walnuts. On rest days, calories drop to about 17 and carbs to about 1.5 grams per pound; keep your protein and fat intakes roughly the same. And make sure you eat frequently, approximately every three hours. (These numbers are based on a 180-pound man.)

Sample Workout Day 1	Sample Workout Day 2	Sample rest Day
Breakfast 1 (upon waking)	**Breakfast 1 (upon waking)**	**Breakfast 1 (upon waking)**
2 scoops whey protein	2 scoops whey protein	2 scoops whey protein
1 apple	1 apple	1 apple
Breakfast 2	**Breakfast 2**	**Breakfast 2**
3 large eggs	3 large eggs	3 large eggs
1 cup oatmeal	2 slices sprouted bread	1 cup oatmeal
1 cup green tea	1 cup green tea	1 cup green tea
Morning Snack	**Morning Snack**	**Morning Snack**
8 oz. plain Greek yogurt	8 oz. plain Greek yogurt	8 oz. plain Greek yogurt
½ cup blueberries	1 oz. walnuts	½ cup blueberries
Lunch	1 oz. dark chocolate	**Lunch**
4 slices sprouted bread	**Lunch**	4 slices sprouted bread
1 can (5 oz.) salmon	1 cup quinoa	1 can (5 oz.) salmon
2 cups spinach	5 oz. shrimp	2 cups spinach
1 cup red bell pepper	1 cup broccoli	1 cup red bell pepper
1 Tbsp. olive oil	1 cup green tea	1 Tbsp. olive oil
1 cup green tea	**Preworkout**	1 cup black coffee
Preworkout	1 cup black coffee	**Midafternoon Snack**
1 cup black coffee	1 scoop whey protein	1 scoop whey protein
1 scoop whey protein	1 cup oatmeal	1 cup milk
1 apple	**Postworkout**	1 oz. dark chocolate
Postworkout	1 scoop whey protein	**Dinner**
1 scoop whey protein	1 cup milk	6 oz. chicken breast
1 cup milk	1 large baked potato	1 cup quinoa
1 large baked potato	**Dinner**	1 cup broccoli
1 oz. dark chocolate	5 oz. grass-fed beef, loin cut	5 oz. red wine
Dinner	½ cup black beans	**Bedtime Snack**
6 oz. chicken breast	2 cups spinach	8 oz. low-fat (1%) cottage cheese
1 cup quinoa	1 cup red bell pepper	1 oz. walnuts
1 cup broccoli	1 Tbsp. olive oil	
5 oz. red wine	5 oz. red wine	**NOTE:** Mix all protein powders according to directions on label.
Bedtime Snack	**Bedtime Snack**	
8 oz. low-fat (1%) cottage cheese	8 oz. low-fat (1%) cottage cheese	
1 oz. walnuts	½ cup blueberries	
Daily Totals: 3,517 calories, 298 g protein, 356 g carbs, 96 g fat	**Daily Totals:** 3,575 calories, 292 g protein, 357 g carbs, 107 g fat	**Daily Totals:** 3,025 calories, 267 g protein, 265 g carbs, 94 g fat

Full Recovery

Work out like an animal day after day with minimal soreness and muscle damage with these nutrition, supplement and physical strategies

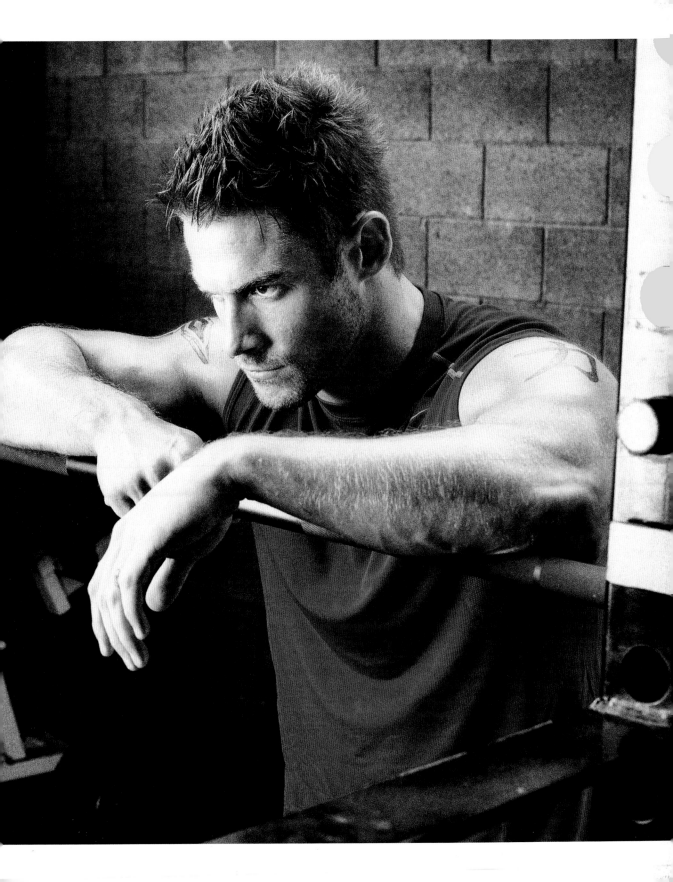

WHEN IT COMES TO TRAINING, MOST of us are guilty of focusing all our energy on our workouts. But like a pilot who can take off but hasn't learned to fly the plane, you're going to get only so far.

Given that you're in the gym two hours a day max (if you train longer and it's not for an Ironman, you're not working hard enough during those 120 minutes) and the other 22 hours are spent recovering, you should focus some energy on ensuring proper recovery. Remember, you don't actually grow in the gym; you break down muscle. It's after the workout that growth and strength gains occur. So if you're not taking time to maximize your recovery efforts, here's some info for you.

WHAT IS RECOVERY?

Recovery begins the second you complete your last rep and can last for days, depending on how hard you trained and how much damage the muscle fibers sustained. Muscles need to recover on two levels: metabolic and structural.

Metabolic recovery involves replenishing muscle fuels such as glycogen, the storage form of carbs; adenosine triphosphate (ATP), the major energy currency of all cells; and creatine phosphate (CP). ATP promotes muscle contractions and is stored in muscles. The body can also break down glycogen to get ATP. Creatine forms CP in muscle cells, which is then used during weight training to create more ATP. When you train at a high intensity, ATP breaks down faster than it can be synthesized.

Structural recovery involves rebuilding muscle-fiber proteins that get damaged during intense workouts. Further damage is caused by free radicals, and some researchers hypothesize that they're responsible for even more damage than mechanical overload. Muscle comprises mostly water, and water is lost through sweat and exhalation, so muscle cells need adequate hydration for fullness and size.

It'd take much longer than a single book chapter to cover all the tissues and systems that need to recuperate after intense exercise, so we'll mention just one: the nervous system. Intense exercise can deplete neurotransmitters such as acetylcholine, dopamine and norepinephrine. These chemicals facilitate communication in the brain, and between the brain and muscles. When they're depleted, cognitive and physical performance suffer. But proper recovery tactics and smart supplementation can restore these precious chemicals.

How you optimize your recovery can make all the difference in gym progress. To help you get back to 100% as quickly as possible, utilize the following recovery windows. For each window we provide nutritional and physical components to enhance your recovery and results.

RECOVERY DON'TS

Don't waste your time on the following methods. Not only have they been shown not to enhance recovery but some may even hinder recovery and growth.

NSAIDs Nonsteroidal anti-inflammatory drugs like ibuprofen are what many guys reach for when they're sore or injured. But using these drugs, which inhibit the inflammatory process that typically ensues after a brutal workout, can be counterproductive. Sure, they'll blunt muscle pain, but research shows they can also inhibit muscle-protein synthesis.

ACUPUNCTURE Acupuncture has been found to alleviate pain resulting from certain medical conditions, but it doesn't enhance muscle recovery.

HYPERBARIC OXYGEN You probably don't have access to a chamber that administers 100% oxygen at environmental pressures greater than one atmosphere, but don't worry: Research shows this technique isn't effective at enhancing muscle recovery and may even increase muscle pain.

MASSAGE We can't blame you for wanting to get a massage. Research shows it won't do much good for true muscle recovery, but it can reduce muscle pain and feel really good.

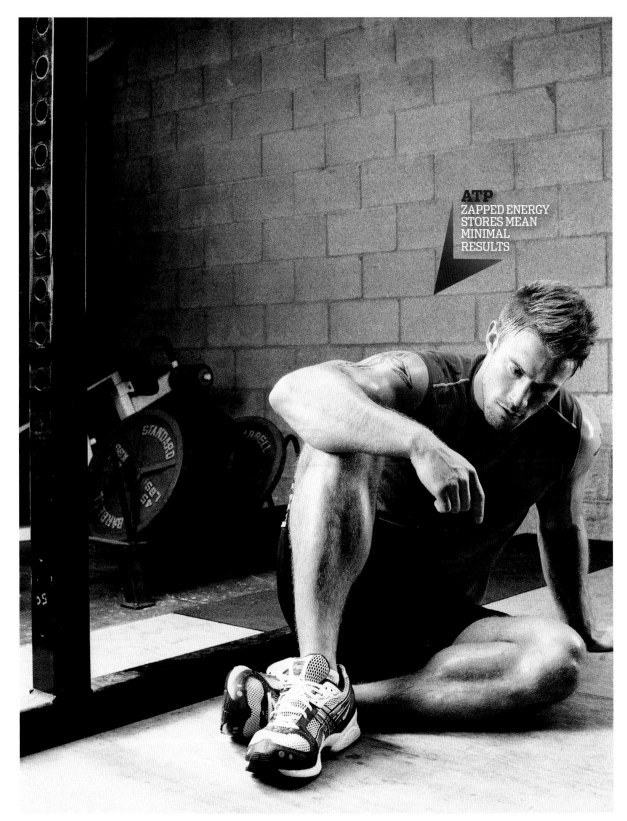

ATP
ZAPPED ENERGY
STORES MEAN
MINIMAL
RESULTS

Before the Workout

ALTHOUGH RECOVERY TECHNICALLY STARTS POSTWORKOUT, YOU CAN PREPARE BEFORE TRAINING.

SUPPLEMENT/NUTRITIONAL RECOVERY

By now it should be second nature to consume a whey protein shake and slow-digesting carbs within 30 minutes preworkout. But these nutrients also improve recovery after you put down the weights. Whey protein limits the amount of muscle that breaks down during the workout while carbs blunt levels of the catabolic hormone cortisol, which increases muscle breakdown.

One great preworkout carb source is tart cherry juice. A study from the University of Vermont (Burlington) reported that subjects who drank 12 ounces of CherryPharm tart cherry juice daily for four days before and after performing a muscle-damaging negative-rep biceps workout experienced almost no strength loss and little muscle pain, while subjects taking a placebo experienced a more than 20% drop in muscle strength and significantly more muscle pain. The cherry juice likely had this effect because of its rich supply of antioxidants, which decrease muscle breakdown and the free-radical onslaught during and after a workout.

Taking branched-chain amino acids (BCAAs) preworkout preserves muscular protein levels and mitigates muscle damage. BCAAs can also keep cortisol levels low. In one study subjects performed intense cycling, and those supplementing with BCAAs were found to have cortisol levels that weren't even half the level of those taking a placebo. Creatine supplementation before a workout can help limit the depletion of ATP and CP during training. Researchers from the University of Connecticut (Storrs) found that taking carnitine inhibits muscle damage following a squat workout. Less damage means more intact receptors to which hormones can bind, instigating muscle recovery and growth.

Exercise Science Writer David Barr, CSCS, CISSN, suggests consuming a fish-oil supplement and whole-food meal sometime before your first rep. "Commonly referred to as fish oil, essential fatty acids (EFAs) become incorporated into cell membranes such as nerve cells. These key fats not only are anchor points for hormone receptors, but they also improve the body's ability to deal with stress and inflammation. This means elevated EFA levels can reduce recovery time by mitigating the inflammatory response," he says.

In addition to these supplements, try green tea extract before workouts. Researchers from Baylor

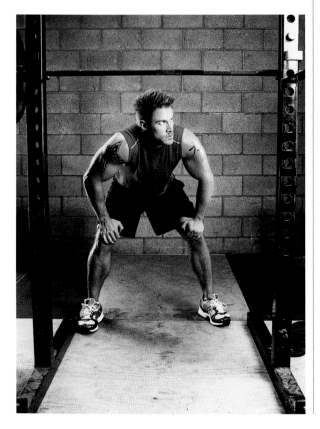

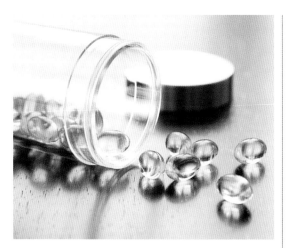

University (Waco, Texas) reported that subjects taking 1,200 mg of epigallocatechin gallate (EGCG) daily for two weeks before a negative-rep leg workout experienced less muscle soreness and damage.

Lastly, consider supplementing with the amino acid tyrosine, which may help boost levels of dopamine and norepinephrine.

RECOVER NOW: At your last whole-food preworkout meal, take 1–2 grams of fish oil. An hour before training, take 500–1,000 mg of green tea extract standardized for EGCG and 2–4 grams of tyrosine. Within 30 minutes before workouts, consume 20 grams of whey protein and 20–40 grams of slow-digesting carbs such as tart cherry juice. Also take 5–10 grams of BCAAs, 3–5 grams of creatine, 1–2 grams of acetyl-L-carnitine and another 1–2 grams of carnitine in the form of L-carnitine, glycine propionyl-L-carnitine or L-carnitine L-tartrate. Be sure to mix your shake in about 20 ounces of water.

PHYSICAL RECOVERY

A warm-up that raises your body temperature is critical to recovery and growth. UK researchers found that when subjects trained in a cold environment, their growth hormone levels were less than half of what they were when they trained in a warm environment. Having elevated GH levels promotes recovery and muscle growth.

RECOVER NOW: Static stretching (reach and hold) is no longer the preferred warm-up. Dynamic stretching — calisthenic-type movements such as arm circles, toe touches and bodyweight walking lunges — is now the superior method. Not only is this a great way to boost body temperature but it also enhances power and strength during a workout.

Another way to warm up is to sit in a sauna or whirlpool for 15–20 minutes. In a 2007 Australian study, subjects had one arm exposed to heat before a negative-rep biceps workout. The heated arm incurred significantly less muscle damage and recovered more quickly than the unheated arm.

During the Workout

WHAT YOU DO DURING YOUR WORKOUT CAN MAKE OR BREAK YOUR RECOVERY.

SUPPLEMENT/NUTRITIONAL RECOVERY

Sip on a caffeinated energy drink to boost your workout performance; caffeine jacks up energy and strength but also has recovery benefits. A 2007 study from the University of Georgia (Athens) reported that subjects taking caffeine before eccentric (negative) contractions in a leg workout experienced less muscle pain and lost less strength than those taking a placebo. In addition, caffeine has been found to restore more than 65% of muscle glycogen levels compared to when carbs are consumed alone.

RECOVER NOW: Try an energy drink that supplies 200–400 mg of caffeine during your workout or take a caffeine pill within an hour of training. Always make sure to drink 5–10 ounces of fluid every 15 minutes.

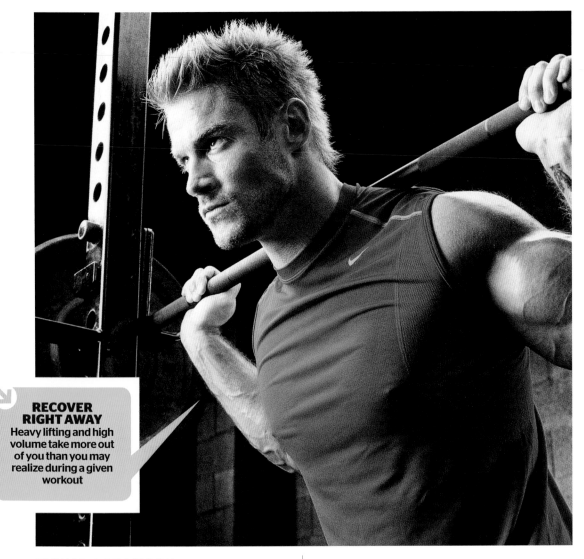

RECOVER RIGHT AWAY
Heavy lifting and high volume take more out of you than you may realize during a given workout

PHYSICAL RECOVERY

One training method that has been shown to enhance recovery and minimize soreness is called cardioacceleration. Researchers from the University of California at Santa Cruz had trained athletes perform a nine-week whole-body weight-training program that utilized slow reps to accentuate muscle damage. The group that performed cardioacceleration — which included a 20-minute warm-up to reach 60%–85% of their max heart rates and 30–60 seconds of cardio between sets to stay in that range — experienced significantly less muscle soreness compared to the group training normally. The UCSC scientists suggested that subjects' higher heart rates increased blood flow to their muscles, which supplied more glucose, amino acids and oxygen.

RECOVER NOW: Instead of resting between sets as you normally do, perform 30–60 seconds of intense cardio. If you don't want to lose your workout station by hopping on a bike or sprinting outdoors, simply jump-rope, do jumping jacks or run in place.

Immediately After the Workout

AS SOON AS YOUR LAST REP IS FINISHED, IT'S TIME TO START THE REAL RECOVERY PROCESS.

SUPPLEMENT/NUTRITIONAL RECOVERY

Just as you know you need to consume protein and carbs before the workout, it's imperative that you also take in both immediately afterward. A study published in the *Journal of Applied Physiology* showed that Marines in basic training who supplemented with a post-exercise protein/carb/fat mixture experienced less muscle pain, and fewer injuries, infections and episodes of heat illness than those eating just carbs and fat, and those who ate nothing post-exercise.

The protein should include whey for speedy delivery to your muscles. Consider whey hydrolysate protein because it breaks down into smaller fragments and absorbs more quickly and easily. A 2006 study from Australia found that subjects consuming a whey hydrolysate product immediately after a negative-rep leg workout regained all their leg strength after two hours, while subjects receiving whey protein isolate or casein protein were found to be weaker than their baseline tests.

Also consider mixing soy protein into your postworkout shake. Research has shown that soy provides better antioxidant protection and reduces postworkout muscle damage even more than whey does. A recent study from the Netherlands reported that subjects taking soy protein experienced a more than 200% increase in GH levels compared to those taking a placebo.

Fast-digesting carbs are best at this time because they spike insulin, which drives more of the protein's glucose and amino acids into muscle cells for better recovery and growth. Also go with another dose of BCAAs, creatine, carnitine and vitamin E, which works with the EFAs to protect your muscles from oxidative damage.

RECOVER NOW: Within 30 minutes postworkout, take 20–30 grams of whey (hydrolysates are preferred) with 10–20 grams of soy protein isolate and 40–80 grams of fast-digesting carbs such as Vitargo or a sports drink. Also get in another 5–10 grams of BCAAs, 3–5 grams of creatine, 1–2 grams of carnitine and 400–800 IU of vitamin E. Mix your protein in 20–32 ounces of water.

PHYSICAL RECOVERY

A Finnish study from the Research Institute for Olympic Sports (Jyväskylä) reported that track and field athletes receiving warm underwater therapy three times a week after intense training experienced greater muscle recovery compared to when they did the same training without the therapy.

Another effective water treatment called contrast therapy alternates between hot and cold tubs. Two recent studies from the Australian Institute of Sport (Canberra) demonstrated that contrast water therapy not only reduced muscle soreness in athletes but also enhanced recovery and hastened the return of muscle strength and power after a negative-rep leg workout. The same researchers reported in a 2008 issue of the *International Journal of Sports Medicine* that athletes following a five-day cycling training program and receiving contrast water therapy experienced improved recovery and were better able to maintain performance levels.

RECOVER NOW: Consider stepping into a hot tub for about 20 minutes three times per week or employ water contrast therapy right after your workout. Since it might be hard to find a cold tub, use an ice pack. Ice your muscles for one minute, then immediately submerge in the hot water (about 100 degrees F) for one minute. Alternate for 14–20 minutes.

Chapter 15

Later That Day

FOR THE REST OF THE DAY, THINK ABOUT NUTRITIONAL AND PHYSICAL EFFORTS THAT'LL ENHANCE YOUR RECOVERY.

SUPPLEMENT/NUTRITIONAL RECOVERY

An hour (no longer than two) after your postworkout shake, consume a whole-food meal that consists of easily digested protein sources such as fish, eggs or lean poultry, as well as slow-digesting carbohydrates such as sweet potatoes, oatmeal or other whole-grain products (whole-wheat breads or brown rice). All other whole-food meals that day should follow these guidelines.

RECOVER NOW: Shoot for 40–60 grams of protein and 40–80 grams of whole-food carbs. Also consider another 1–2-gram dose of fish oil.

PHYSICAL RECOVERY

Even though physical activity may be the furthest

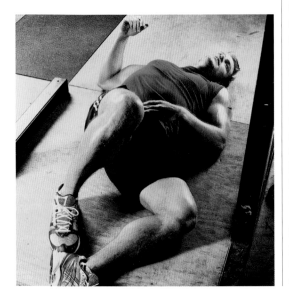

thing from your mind, taking a yoga class could prove helpful. One study published in a 2004 issue of the *Journal of Strength & Conditioning Research* reported that a yoga session following a muscle-damaging leg workout significantly helped reduce muscle pain. Other studies have found that yoga moves can lower levels of the catabolic hormone cortisol.

RECOVER NOW: Attend a few yoga classes each week to help keep cortisol in check and improve your flexibility.

That Night

SLEEP IS A MAJOR FACTOR IN PROPER RECOVERY. ENSURING THAT YOU GET NOT ONLY ADEQUATE BUT QUALITY SLEEP IS VITAL.

SUPPLEMENT/NUTRITIONAL RECOVERY

We used to avoid eating at night for fear of getting fat. Now we know better. Getting 7–9 hours of sleep each night is necessary, but it's also a multihour fast that can wreak havoc on your hard-earned muscle mass. That's why we always recommend drinking a casein shake right before bed. This very slow-digesting milk protein provides a steady stream of amino acids for up to seven hours. Another supplement to consider at bedtime is ZMA, a combination of zinc, magnesium aspartate and vitamin B_6. One study found that athletes who supplemented with ZMA before bed had increased anabolic hormone levels, including free testosterone and insulinlike growth factor-1. ZMA can also improve sleep quality.

RECOVER NOW: Go with one dose of ZMA (most products provide 30 mg of zinc, 450 mg of magnesium aspartate and 11 mg of B_6 per dose) on an empty stomach about one hour before bed. Immediately before bed, have 20–40 grams of casein protein, preferably micellar casein, which is the slowest-digesting form.

PHYSICAL RECOVERY

You don't want to be too physical before bed, as an elevated heart rate and body temperature can upset your ability to relax. You also want to avoid bright lights, which can offset your production of melatonin — a hormone that encourages deep sleep. One recent study reported that subjects with sleep complaints slept better after listening to classical music. If you have problems sleeping, try listening to relaxing music before bed.

RECOVER NOW: About an hour before bed, dim the lights, and turn off the TV and computer monitors. While lying in bed, listen to relaxing music.

The Next Day

JUST BECAUSE THE DAY ENDS DOESN'T MEAN RECOVERY HAS TO. THESE TIPS WILL KEEP YOUR RESULTS ON TRACK.

SUPPLEMENT/NUTRITIONAL RECOVERY

Even though you took casein before bed, your body will be in a catabolic state when you wake up. It's looking for aminos to convert into glucose for fuel, and your muscles are prime targets. Although testosterone is high when you wake, so is the T-blunting hormone cortisol. Getting some fast protein and carbs will stop the breakdown of muscle protein and lower cortisol levels. Also consider BCAAs, which will help prevent muscle protein breakdown.

RECOVER NOW: As soon as you wake up, get 20–40 grams of whey protein, 5–10 grams of BCAAs and

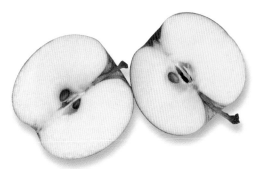

about 40 grams of carbs. Fruit is a good source of carbohydrate for this first meal because the fructose will go straight to the liver to restock the glycogen lost during the night. Restoring liver glycogen levels stops the body from attacking your muscles for fuel.

PHYSICAL RECOVERY

You probably planned to go to the gym today to train different body parts, but we suggest you also train the same muscle group as yesterday. This is known scientifically as active recovery or a feeder workout. Research has shown that performing a few light sets can decrease muscle soreness and increase force recovery because it stimulates nutritive blood flow to damaged muscle fibers.

RECOVER NOW: The studies on active recovery used about 50 easily performed, submaximal contractions. The day after a brutal workout, perform one set of one of the same exercises for 10–15 reps using a weight with which you could normally complete about 50 reps. Shoot for 40–60 reps for each muscle group.

GOING BACK FOR MORE

The most obvious question now is, how long should you allow a muscle to recover before training it again (excluding feeder workouts)? Studies show the answer depends on the individual. Most studies concur, however, that 48 hours is sufficient recovery for most subjects, with some needing 72–96 hours. How do you know where you fall? Visit muscleandfitness.com to learn how to test your muscle recovery.

Exercise**Index**

Abs→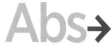

CABLE CRUNCH

Kneel a couple of feet in front of a cable weight stack with a rope attached to a high-pulley cable. Grasp the ends of the rope and hold them on either side of your head. Begin slightly bent over, then contract your abs to lower your torso toward the floor. As with the crunch, the range of motion here is slight; your head shouldn't reach the floor. The key is a full contraction of the abs.

STANDING CABLE CRUNCH →

Stand a few feet in front of a cable weight stack with a rope attached to a high pulley. Grasp the rope and hold it around your neck. Begin bent over, then contract your abs to lower your torso toward the floor in a crunching motion. Squeeze your abs for a count, then slowly return to the start position.

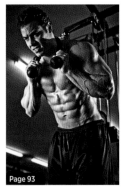

Page 93

CRUNCH

Lie faceup on the floor with your knees and hips bent about 90 degrees, feet in the air and either cross your arms over your chest or place your hands lightly behind your head. Contract your abs to lift your shoulder blades off the floor, then lower slowly. The range of motion is very short; the goal is to press your lower back into the floor to bring your sternum closer to your pelvis.

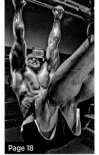

Page 18

← HANGING LEG RAISE

Hang from a pull-up bar or vertical bench with your legs straight and perpendicular to the floor. Keeping your knees extended but not locked out, raise your legs in front of you until they're parallel to the floor. Concentrate on contracting your abs, not your hip flexors, throughout the movement. Slowly lower your legs back to the hanging position.

REVERSE CRUNCH

Lie faceup on the floor with your hands at your sides or under your glutes. Begin with your legs extended and your feet a few inches off the floor, suspended in the air to put tension on your abs. Contract your abs to slowly raise your legs, keeping them straight, until they're roughly perpendicular to the floor. (As with the hanging leg raise, your abs are the focus, not your hip flexors.) Slowly lower your legs back to the start position without letting your feet touch the floor.

ONE-ARM KETTLE BELL CRUNCH ↓

Lie faceup on the floor with your knees bent, holding a kettlebell in one hand above your face. With the kettlebell in position, contract your abs to raise your shoulders off the floor. Repeat for reps, then switch sides.

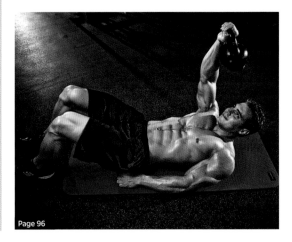

Page 96

MACHINE CRUNCH

Sit inside a crunch machine with your arms across the pad. With your feet flat on the floor, flex your abs to crunch forward, moving the pad toward your knees. Squeeze and hold, then return to the start position. Don't allow the weight plates to touch between reps.

SIT-UP

Lie faceup on the floor with your knees bent 90 degrees and your feet secured underneath a stable structure with your hands either behind your head or your arms crossed over your chest. Contract your abs to initiate a full sit-up, then slowly return to the start position. Sit-ups can also be performed while holding a weight plate against your chest.

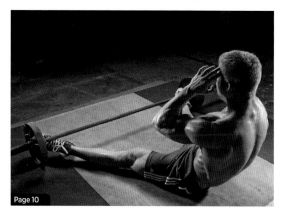
Page 10

SPREAD-EAGLE SIT-UP ↑

Load a bar with a 25-pound plate on each side and place it on the floor. Sit down and hook your feet under the bar, keeping your legs straight and spread as wide as possible. Lie back on the floor. Crunch your torso up by bending at the waist and hips. Lower back down until your shoulder blades touch the floor.

INCLINE SIT-UP

Lie back on an incline sit-up board or decline bench with your feet secured under the pad and your hands either behind your head or your arms crossed over your chest. Begin with the back of your shoulders on the bench. Contract your abs to initiate a full sit-up, then slowly return to the start position.

PLANK

Assume push-up position, only with the pinky side of your forearms (the ulna bones) on the floor. (A padded surface may be preferred for comfort.) You should be supported by only your forearms and toes, with your body in a straight line from head to feet, head facing the floor. Hold this position for a length of time. The key is to keep your core tight to avoid letting your pelvis drop toward the floor. As you get stronger on this static exercise, increase the amount of time you hold the plank.

DUMBBELL SIDE BEND

Stand with your feet shoulder-width apart, holding a dumbbell in your right hand with that arm hanging at your side. Bend at the waist to the left to lower yourself. When you feel a stretch in your side, reverse the motion by contracting your obliques to return to the standing position. Repeat all reps to that side, then switch sides.

RUSSIAN TWIST

Lie faceup on the floor and extend your arms overhead, grasping something secure. Keeping your shoulders on the floor but elevating your hips slightly, extend your legs above you and slowly lower them to the floor on the right side. Reverse and touch the floor on the left side. Add resistance by holding a medicine ball between your knees.

BARBELL ROLLOUT ↓

Place a barbell on the floor and kneel behind it with your knees hip-width apart and your toes on the floor. Lean forward to grasp the bar with a shoulder-width or narrower, overhand grip. Keeping your arms straight, roll the barbell forward, using your abs to hold your body rigid, until your arms are fully extended. Contract your abs to reverse the motion.

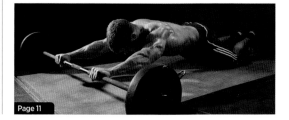
Page 11

Back→

PULL-UP →

Take a wide grip on a pull-up bar (hands outside shoulder width) and start in a hanging position, arms fully extended. Pull yourself up explosively by contracting your lats until your chin clears the bar. Slowly lower yourself to the start position.

Page 83

LAT PULLDOWN

Adjust the seat of the machine so your knees fit snugly under the pads. Grasp the bar outside shoulder width, arms fully extended overhead. Contract your lats to pull the bar past your chin, squeeze your back muscles and slowly return the weight to the start position.

REVERSE-GRIP LAT PULLDOWN

Sit in a lat pulldown machine and grasp the bar with a reverse (palms facing you), shoulder-width grip, maintaining an erect posture with your arms extended above you. Contract your lats to pull the bar to your upper chest, bringing your elbows straight down and as far behind you as possible. Squeeze your shoulder blades together at the bottom, then slowly return to the start position.

BARBELL BENT-OVER ROW ↓

Stand holding a barbell with a shoulder-width, overhand grip. Bend your knees slightly and lean forward at the waist so your torso is roughly 45 degrees to the floor; maintain this position throughout. Start with your arms extended, hanging straight down, and bend your elbows to pull the bar into your midsection. At the top of the move, squeeze your shoulder blades together for a count to fully contract your back muscles, then slowly return to the start position. For a reverse-grip bent-over row, the technique is the same, except that your hands will hold the bar in an underhand (supinated) grip.

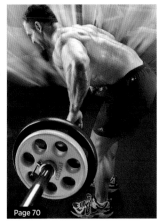

Page 70

SMITH MACHINE BENT-OVER ROW

Stand in a Smith machine and grasp the bar with a shoulder-width, overhand grip. Bend your knees slightly and bend over at your waist so your torso is 45 degrees to parallel to the floor. Start with your arms extended, hanging straight down, and pull the bar to your stomach. Squeeze your shoulder blades together at the top, then slowly return the bar to the start position.

SEATED CABLE ROW

Sit on the bench at a cable-row station with your feet flat on the platform. Bend at your waist to grasp the attachment with both hands and sit upright (back flat, not bowed), arms extended in front of you. Bend your elbows to pull the handle straight toward your midsection by contracting your back muscles; de-emphasize the amount of work your biceps do to keep maximal tension on your back. When your hands reach your abs, squeeze your shoulder blades together and hold before slowly returning to the start.

STANDING CABLE ROW

Stand in front of a cable stack with your feet shoulder-width apart and grasp a straight bar attached to the low pulley with an overhand grip and your arms extended. Keeping your knees slightly bent, lean forward at your waist until your torso is roughly parallel to the floor. Without raising your upper body, pull the bar to your abdomen, bringing your elbows high and above the level of your back. Squeeze your shoulder blades together, then lower the bar back to the start position. This exercise can also be performed using a rope attachment, where your palms face each other.

T-BAR ROW

With your feet flat on the platform of a T-bar row apparatus and your knees slightly bent, grasp the bar with your hands close together and extend your arms toward the floor. Pull the weight toward your midsection by contracting your middle back muscles. When you've pulled the bar as far up as possible (as far as the weight plates will allow), slowly lower it back to the arms-extended position.

ONE-ARM DUMBBELL ROW ↓

Place one knee and the same-side hand on a flat bench, and bent over at the waist. Keep your other foot on the floor beside the bench and hold a dumbbell in the same-side hand, letting it hang straight down. Pull the weight to

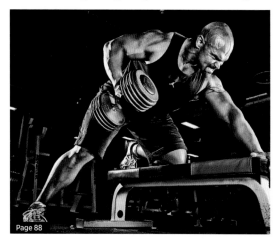

Page 88

your side, keeping your elbow in close. Pull your elbow as high as you can, squeezing your shoulder blades together for a full contraction, then lower.

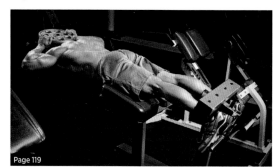

Page 119

WEIGHTED BACK EXTENSION →

Grab a weight plate and secure your feet in a back-extension apparatus. Allow your upper body to hang freely, keeping your

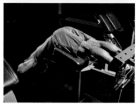

back flat. Hold the plate behind your head, squeeze your glutes and slowly raise your torso until your body forms a straight line. Slowly return to the start.

RACK PULL

Inside a power rack, place the bar on the safeties just below knee level and grasp the bar just outside your legs. Keep the bar flush against your legs. With your abs tight, back flat, arms straight and chest up, press through your feet to raise the bar, dragging it up your quads until you're standing. Lower the bar along the same path, allowing it to settle on the safety bars, then repeat.

STRAIGHT-ARM PULLDOWN

Stand facing a cable stack and attach a straight bar or rope handle to a high-pulley cable. Grasp the attachment with both hands, and begin with your arms extended in front of you and your hands at roughly head level. (Make sure the weight isn't resting on the stack.) Contract your lats to pull the attachment toward your thighs, keeping your elbows extended to isolate your back muscles.

Biceps/ Forearms→

BARBELL CURL ↓

Stand holding a barbell with an underhand grip in front of your thighs, arms extended and knees slightly bent to prevent putting pressure on your lower back. Keeping your elbows at your sides, curl the weight as high as you can. Squeeze your biceps for a count at the top, then slowly return the bar to the start position.

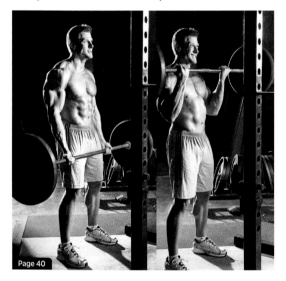

Page 40

DUMBBELL CURL →

Hold a pair of dumbbells outside your thighs, palms up. Using one arm at a time, curl the weight toward your shoulder without swinging it or rolling your shoulder, making sure your upper arm is locked at your side. Squeeze your biceps at the top, then slowly lower to the start.

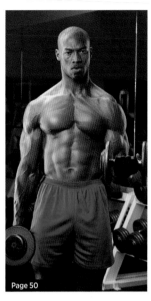

Page 50

CABLE CURL

Stand facing a cable stack, holding a bar attached to a low pulley with an underhand grip, arms extended. Contract your biceps to curl the bar toward your chest, keeping your elbows at your sides. Hold and squeeze at the top, then slowly return the bar along the same path.

PREACHER CURL

Sit at a preacher bench and adjust the seat so the top of the pad fits snugly under your armpits. Grasp a straight bar or EZ-bar with a shoulder-width grip, arms extended but not locked out. Keeping your upper arms flush against the pad, curl the weight as high as you can and squeeze the contraction. Lower the bar under control, again stopping just shy of locking out your elbows.

DUMBBELL INCLINE CURL

Adjust an incline bench to 45–60 degrees and lie faceup on the bench with your feet flat on the floor. Hold a pair of dumbbells with your arms hanging straight down, palms forward. Keeping your shoulders back and upper arms fixed perpendicular to the floor, curl the dumbbells toward your shoulders. Squeeze your biceps hard at the top before slowly returning to the start position.

DUMBBELL SCOTT CURL

Grasp a pair of dumbbells and lean your chest against the angled side of a preacher bench. Make certain your armpit fits securely over the top of the pad, with your triceps pressed into the flat side of the bench. Place your nonworking hand on the bench for balance and hold the dumbbell straight down toward the floor with a palms-up grip. Curl it in a smooth arc, then squeeze your biceps hard for a count before slowly lowering the dumbbell back to the start position.

MACHINE CURL

Adjust the seat of a curl machine so that the backs of your upper arms are in contact with the pad (not just your elbows). Starting with your arms fully extended, grasp the handles and curl the weight as far as possible. Hold the contraction for a count, then lower to the start position without letting the weight rest on the stack.

CABLE PREACHER CURL

Set a preacher curl bench a couple of feet in front of a cable stack with a straight or EZ-bar attached to the low pulley. Sit and grasp the bar with a shoulder-width grip, arms extended but not locked out. With your upper arms flush against the pad, curl the weight as high as you can and squeeze the contraction. Lower the bar under control, stopping just shy of locking out your elbows.

LYING CABLE CURL

Attach a straight bar to a pulley set approximately halfway up the column (or the high pulley if the cable apparatus doesn't adjust). Lie faceup on the floor or a bench with your head a foot or so away from the stack, your knees bent and your feet flat on the floor. Grasp the bar with a shoulder-width grip and your arms extended straight up. Keeping your upper arms stationary, curl the bar to your forehead. Squeeze your biceps for a count when it reaches your head, then slowly return the bar to the start position.

STANDING ONE-ARM DUMBBELL PREACHER CURL

Stand holding a dumbbell and drape your arm over a preacher bench. Keeping your shoulder down, raise the dumbbell in an arc toward your face. Stop just short of bringing your forearm perpendicular to the floor. Squeeze at the top, then return to the start position.

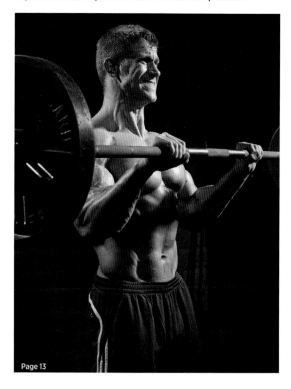

Page 13

BARBELL REVERSE CURL ↑

Grasp a barbell with an overhand, shoulder-width grip and let it hang in front of your thighs. With your elbows close to your sides, bend them to curl the bar toward your shoulders. Return along the same path.

SMITH MACHINE DRAG CURL

Stand in a Smith machine holding the bar in front of your upper thighs with your chest up, shoulders back and eyes focused forward. Pull your elbows back as you curl the bar toward your lower chest. As the name suggests, drag the bar up your torso as high as possible, keeping your elbows behind you. Slowly return the bar along the same path.

Exercise**Index**

BICEPS/FOREARMS →

SEATED BARBELL CURL

Sit on a flat bench with a barbell on your lap and your feet flat on the floor. Grasp the bar with a shoulder-width grip and bend your elbows roughly 90 degrees, keeping your elbows in at your sides. Keeping your upper body stationary (don't lean back), curl the bar as far as possible and squeeze your biceps. Lower the bar back to the start position; don't let it rest on your legs between reps.

POWER-RACK CURL

Set the safety pins of a power rack so the bar rests on them at the bottom of your curl range of motion (where your arms are just shy of full extension). Start with the bar resting on the pins, grasp the bar with a shoulder-width grip (palms facing forward) and keep your elbows in at your sides. Curl the bar, then slowly lower it back to the pins. Begin every rep with the bar on the pins to eliminate all momentum at the beginning of each curl.

HAMMER CURL

Stand holding a pair of dumbbells at your sides with your wrists in a neutral position (palms facing in). Flex your elbows to curl both dumbbells without turning your palms up — keep them neutral. Squeeze your biceps and forearms at the top, then lower the weights to the start position. Hammer curls can also be performed at a cable station using a rope attachment with the pulley set at the lowest position.

LOW-CABLE TOWEL CURL

Stand facing a cable stack and drape a towel around an attachment fixed to a low-pulley cable so the ends of the towel point up, similar to a rope attachment. Grasp the ends of the towel and extend your arms in front of you, hands in front of your thighs and palms facing each other. Contract your biceps to curl the towel toward your chest, keeping your elbows at your sides. Hold and squeeze at the top, then slowly return the bar along the same path.

RACK-SUPPORTED WRIST ROLLER ↗

Set the bar in a power rack to about chest level. Holding a wrist roller with a weight attached, rest your forearms against on bar. Grasp the handle with your left hand and slide your right hand behind the handle

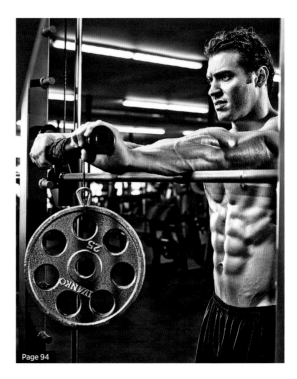

Page 94

by hyperextending your wrist, then regrip. Repeat this "pushing" sequence, alternating hands until the weight is as high as it can go. Lower the weight steadily and repeat in the opposite direction in a "pulling" sequence. That's one rep.

BARBELL WRIST CURL

Straddle a flat bench with your feet flat on the floor. Hold a straight bar with a palms-up grip and rest the backs of your forearms on the bench so your hands hang off the end. Start with your wrists extended so your knuckles point toward the floor and the bar rests on only your fingers. Flex your wrists by contracting your forearm muscles to raise the bar; the range of motion is only a few inches. Squeeze your forearms for 1–2 counts at the top, then slowly return to the wrists-extended position.

BARBELL REVERSE WRIST CURL

Sit at the end of a flat bench, holding a barbell with a narrow, overhand grip. Allow your forearms to rest on your quads, with only your hands extending past your knees. Curl the bar, squeezing your forearms, then return to the start position.

Chest→

BENCH PRESS ↓

Lie faceup on a flat bench with a rack and grasp the barbell just outside shoulder width. Carefully lift the bar off the rack and lower it toward your chest. Lightly touch the bar to your lower pecs, then forcefully press it up to an arms-extended position without locking out your elbows. The bar should be directly above your face. The path of motion here is a slight backward arc rather than a straight line up from the lower pecs.

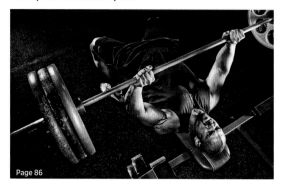
Page 86

SMITH MACHINE BENCH PRESS

Position a flat bench in the center of a Smith machine. Set the safeties low enough so that when you lower the bar, it touches your lower pecs. Lie faceup on the bench and grasp the bar outside shoulder width. Lower the bar to your chest under control, then press it back up explosively.

FLAT-BENCH DUMBBELL PRESS

Lie on a flat bench and hold a set of dumbbells just above chest level with your palms facing forward and your wrists directly over your elbows. Press the dumbbells up and in toward each other over your mid-chest until your elbows are almost locked out. Bring the weights back down until your elbows form 90-degree angles.

BARBELL INCLINE PRESS

Lie faceup on a bench set to a 45-degree incline with a rack and grasp the bar with a slightly wider than shoulder-width grip. Start with the bar directly above your upper pecs and your arms extended but not locked out. Lower the bar to your chest, then press it up forcefully to the start position.

SMITH MACHINE INCLINE PRESS

Lie on an incline bench set inside a Smith machine and grasp the bar with a shoulder-width, overhand grip. Unrack the bar and hold it directly above your upper chest, then slowly lower the bar. When it reaches your chest, powerfully press the bar back up to the start position.

DUMBBELL INCLINE PRESS

Lie faceup on an adjustable incline bench and start with the dumbbells just outside your shoulders. Press the weights straight above you until your elbows are extended but not locked out. Slowly return to the start position.

BARBELL DECLINE PRESS

Lie faceup on a decline bench with a rack and grasp a barbell with a wider than shoulder-width grip. Unrack the weight, begin with your arms extended above you and lower the bar to your chest. After lightly touching the bar to your lower pecs, press it up to the start position without locking out your elbows.

DUMBBELL DECLINE PRESS

Lie faceup on a decline bench with your feet secured beneath the pads and start with the dumbbells just outside your lower pecs. Press the weights straight up until your elbows are extended but not locked out. Slowly return to the start position.

Exercise**Index**

CHEST →

SMITH MACHINE DECLINE PRESS

Position a decline bench symmetrically in a Smith machine so that when you lower the bar, it touches your lower pecs. Lie faceup on the bench and grasp the bar outside shoulder width. Lower the bar to your chest under control, then press it back up explosively, keeping your elbows out.

MACHINE CHEST PRESS

Adjust the seat of the machine so that when you grasp the handles your hands are at lower chest level. Sit with your back flat against the pad and begin with the weight off the stack to keep tension on the pecs. Press the weight away from you by contracting your chest muscles and extending your arms until your elbows are fully extended but not locked out. Keep your eyes facing forward throughout.

DIP

Start by holding yourself between the bars of a dip apparatus with your arms extended. Lower yourself under control until your upper arms are parallel to the floor and you feel a good stretch in your chest, then push with your chest and triceps to lift yourself back to the start position. To do weighted dips, hang a weight plate or dumbbell from a chain attached to a lifting belt.

PULLOVER

Place your upper back across a flat bench with your knees bent and your feet on the floor in front of you for balance. Hold one end of a dumbbell with both hands, the other end hanging down, and your arms extended with the weight over your chest. With only a slight bend in your elbows, lower the dumbbell in an arc beyond your head until you feel a stretch in your chest and lats. Pull the weight back to the start position by contracting your pecs. Pullovers can also be done on an incline or decline bench and/or with a barbell using the same technique to train the muscles from a slightly different angle.

CABLE CROSSOVER ↗

Stand in the middle of a two-sided cable station with D-handles attached to both high-pulley cables. Begin with your arms extended out to your sides and elbows slightly bent. Step forward to make sure the weights aren't resting

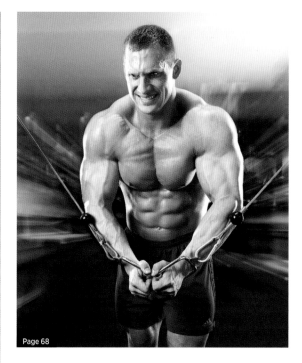

Page 68

on the stacks, then contract your pecs to pull your hands together, maintaining the slight bend in your elbows. At the end of the motion, cross your hands and squeeze your pecs for a count.

FLAT-BENCH DUMBBELL FLYE

Lie faceup on the bench with your feet flat on the floor. Hold a dumbbell in each hand with a neutral grip and extend your arms above your chest. Bend your elbows slightly. Slowly lower the dumbbells in a wide arc out to your sides. Keep your elbows locked in the slightly bent position throughout the range of motion. Stop when your elbows reach shoulder level, then contract your pecs to reverse the motion and return to the start position.

FLAT-BENCH CABLE FLYE

Place a flat bench equidistant between two low-pulley cables. Grasp the two D-handles attached to the cables and lie faceup on the bench. Keeping your arms slightly bent, pull the handles in front of you, as if you were hugging a barrel. Squeeze your pecs together when your hands are above your torso, then lower the handles back down, stopping when your upper arms are level with the bench.

DUMBBELL BUTT-END FLYE ↓

Lie faceup on a bench holding two dumbbells above your chest using a neutral grip, elbows slightly bent. Lower the weights out to your sides in an arc until you feel a stretch in your chest. Return along the same path while rotating your wrists so your palms face you at the top. Touch the ends together and squeeze.

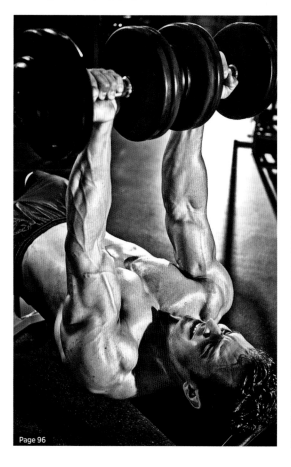

Page 96

DUMBBELL INCLINE FLYE

Lie faceup on an adjustable bench set to 45 degrees, holding a pair of dumbbells over your chest with your arms extended and palms facing each other. With a slight bend in your elbows, lower the weights out in an arc to your sides until you feel a good stretch in your pecs. Contract your muscles to return the dumbbells to the start position, maintaining the slight bend in your elbows throughout.

DECLINE PUSH-UP ↓

Place your hands about shoulder-width apart flat on the floor and your toes up on a bench behind you, keeping your body flat and rigid. Begin with your arms extended, perpendicular to the floor. Bend your elbows to slowly lower yourself to the floor. When your chest reaches a few inches from touching, extend your elbows to forcefully press yourself back up to the start position.

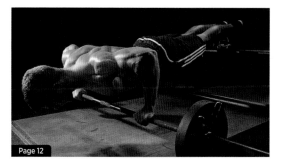

Page 12

BARBELL DECLINE PUSH-UP

With your feet elevated on a bench, get in push-up position with your hands grasping a barbell at approximately shoulder width. Keeping your body straight, bend your elbows to lower your chest to the bar, then push back up to the start.

SVEND PRESS

Stand erect and press two 10-pound plates together in front of your chest with your fingers pointing up. From that position, extend your arms out in front of you as far as you can, maintaining pressure on the plates throughout the move. As you bring the weights back, squeeze your lats and push your chest out to meet the plates.

Legs/ Full Body →

SQUAT (BARBELL AND BODYWEIGHT)

Stand erect holding a barbell across your upper traps. With your feet about shoulder-width apart and head facing forward, push your chest out slightly so your back arches naturally. Squat down with the weight as if to sit in a chair, keeping your feet in full contact with the floor and maintaining the arch in your back. When your thighs reach parallel to the floor, press through your heels, extending your knees and hips to return to standing. A bodyweight squat consists of the same technique without the added weight.

POWER CLEAN

Stand over a loaded barbell on the floor with your shins about an inch from the bar and your feet shoulder-width apart. Squat down to grasp the bar with an overhand grip. With your abs pulled in tight and your entire body tense, perform the following sequence in one fluid motion: Drive explosively through your heels to straighten your knees and bring your hips forward until the bar is at hip level, then immediately pull the bar up to your shoulders and squat under the bar as you catch it on your shoulders with your elbows pointing forward. Extend at the hips and knees to stand straight up keeping a slight bend in your knees and allowing the bar to rest on your upper chest and front delts. Lower the bar back to the floor and repeat.

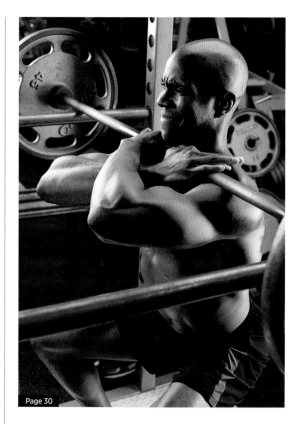
Page 30

BARBELL FRONT SQUAT ↑

Stand inside a power rack with the barbell across your front delts and upper chest. Cross your arms over your chest to build a shelf for the bar, unrack it and step back so you clear the rack. Keep your chest up and back flat, eyes focused forward. With your abs tight, bend your knees and hips as if to sit in a chair until your thighs are well past parallel to the floor. Reverse direction by driving through your heels and pressing your hips forward.

POWER SNATCH

Grasp a light barbell on the floor with your hands well outside shoulder width and your feet about hip width. Bend at the hips and knees, and keep your head and chest up, and your arms fully extended. Initiate the lift as explosively as possible by extending the hips and knees while pulling the bar off the floor, keeping your arms straight. As the bar reaches chest level, duck under it and lift it overhead. Stand up to complete the lift, then return the weight to the floor and repeat. This exercise differs from a regular snatch in that you don't go into a full squat at the bottom — only a quarter squat.

LEG PRESS

Sit on a leg-press machine and place your feet hip- to shoulder-width apart on the foot platform above you. Press the weight up with your legs to the point where your knees are extended but not locked out. Release the machine's safety catches. Lower the weight under control until your knees form 90-degree angles or slightly less. Push the weight back up explosively to the start position, again without locking out your knees.

SMITH MACHINE SQUAT

Stand erect in a Smith machine with the bar set so it rests across your upper back. Your feet are shoulder-width apart, knees slightly bent and toes turned out slightly. Rotate the bar to unrack it. Keeping your eyes focused forward and abs tight, bend at the knees and hips to slowly lower your body, as if to sit in a chair. Pause when your knees reach a 90-degree angle, then forcefully drive through your heels, extending at your hips and knees until you arrive at the standing position.

JUMP SQUAT

Stand with a light barbell resting across your upper traps (as in a standard squat), knees slightly bent with roughly a shoulder-width stance. Keeping your chest up and back flat, squat down until your thighs approach parallel to the floor, then explode up as high as possible, jumping off the floor. Land softly with your knees bent and immediately go into the next rep.

HACK SQUAT

Step inside a hack-squat machine, placing your shoulders and back against the pads, with your feet shoulder-width apart on the platform and your legs extended. Maintain good posture, with your chest up and abs pulled in tight. Unhook the safety bars and bend your knees to slowly

lower yourself until they're past 90 degrees. Pause, then forcefully press yourself up to the start position without locking out your knees at the top.

LEG EXTENSION

Adjust the seat of a leg-extension machine so your lower back is against the seatback and your knees line up with the machine's axis of rotation. Begin with your knees bent 90 degrees and the weight lifted a few inches off the stack. Contract your quads to extend your legs until they're completely straight. Squeeze your quads at the top, then return to the start position.

DEADLIFT ↓

Stand in an open space with a loaded barbell on the floor in front of you, feet hip-width apart. Keeping your back flat and head up, bend your knees and hips to grasp the bar with a shoulder-width, mixed (one palm facing forward, the other backward) grip. This is your start position. Stand up with the bar in one explosive motion by extending your knees and hips. Never round your back. Return under control to the start position, touching the weight to the floor.

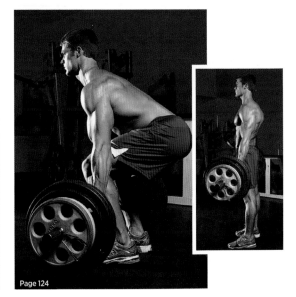

Page 124

LEGS/FULL BODY →

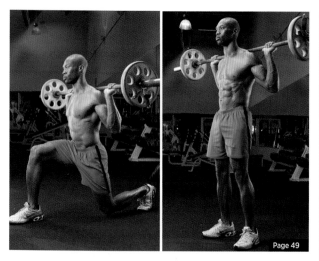

Page 49

LUNGE

Hold a dumbbell in each hand and stand with your feet hip-width apart and your arms down at your sides. (Lunges can also be performed holding a barbell across your upper traps.) Step forward a comfortable stride length with one foot, lift your back heel and lower your back knee toward the floor. When your front thigh is parallel to the floor, press through the heel of your front foot, raising your body straight up to the start position. Step forward with the other foot and repeat. Continue alternating legs until you've completed all the reps for one set. Lunges can also be performed walking, where instead of stepping back to the start position on each rep, you step forward with your back foot so it meets your front foot, gaining ground with each rep.

SMITH MACHINE LUNGE

Stand in a Smith machine with the bar resting across your upper traps and your feet together. Unhook the latches and step a few feet forward with one foot, keeping both legs extended. Bend your front knee and drop your back knee until it's a few inches from touching the floor. (Your front knee shouldn't extend past your toes; if it does, step out farther.) Contract the quad and glute of your front leg to press yourself back up to the standing position. Repeat for reps, then switch legs.

← REVERSE LUNGE

Hold a dumbbell in each hand or a barbell across your upper traps and stand erect with your feet hip-width apart. Step backward with one foot and lower that knee toward the floor; only the ball of your back foot should touch the floor, not the heel. When your front thigh is parallel to the floor, press off your back foot to lift your body back to the start position. Repeat with the opposite leg. Continue alternating legs until you've completed all the reps for one set.

DUMBBELL STEP-UP

Select a bench or box that's 12–18 inches high. Start by standing upright holding dumbbells at your sides, keeping your head up and chest out to maintain proper back alignment. Step up so your entire foot is on the bench, then stand up, pressing into the bench, pulling your trailing leg up. After both feet are on the bench, slowly move your trailing leg back down, emphasizing the negative motion. Maintain proper back alignment during the lift. Alternate legs every rep or do all the reps for one leg, then switch.

GOOD MORNING

Set a light barbell across your upper back/traps and position your feet at shoulder width with your knees slightly bent. With your torso erect and eyes focused ahead, push your glutes back and bend at the waist until your torso is parallel to the floor. Pause deliberately at the bottom before contracting your lower back, glutes and hamstrings to raise your torso back to the start position.

LYING LEG CURL

Adjust the machine so the roller pad rests over the backs of your ankles. Lie facedown and grasp the handles. Start with your legs straight and the weight lifted a few inches off the stack. Bend your knees to curl the roller pad toward your glutes. Squeeze your hamstrings for a count at the top and slowly lower to the start position.

LEG CURL

Adjust the seat so your knees line up with the machine's axis of rotation. Sit squarely in the machine, placing the backs of your ankles on the rollers and securing the pad across your lower quads. Begin with your legs extended, then contract your hamstrings to flex your knees as far as possible. Hold for a count at the bottom, then slowly return to the start position.

ROMANIAN DEADLIFT ↓

Stand upright, holding a barbell in front of your thighs with a shoulder-width grip. With your back flat and knees slightly bent, lean forward at the waist to slide the bar down your legs. Keep your knees slightly bent and your arms straight throughout the movement. When the bar reaches about mid-shin level (how far you can lower it depends on your flexibility), contract your hamstrings and glutes to pull yourself back up to the start position.

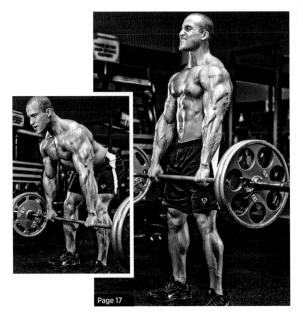

Page 17

SEATED CALF RAISE

Sit and adjust the pads so they fit snugly over your lower thighs. Place the balls of your feet on the platform so your heels are suspended. Release the safety catch and lower your heels below the level of the platform until you feel a stretch in your calves. Extend your ankles to push the pads up as high as you can — you should be almost on

your tiptoes at the top. Squeeze your calves, then lower back down.

DONKEY CALF RAISE

Step into a donkey calf-raise machine and place the balls of your feet on the platform with your upper glutes/lower back secured under the pad provided. Allow your forearms to rest on the arm pads and grasp the handles. Press up onto your toes by contracting your calves, squeeze the contraction and lower your heels as close to the floor as possible.

STANDING CALF RAISE →

Step onto the platform with the balls of your feet so your heels are suspended. Place your shoulders snugly underneath the pads. Drop your heels toward the floor below the level of the platform, keeping your knees slightly bent throughout. Flex your calves to extend your ankles as high as possible. Squeeze your calves 1-2 counts at the top, then lower back to the start position, feeling a stretch at the bottom.

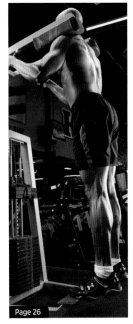

Page 26

DUMBBELL SEATED CALF RAISE

Sit on a seat or the end of a flat bench and place the balls of your feet on a raised surface (like a wood block) so your heels are suspended. Place a pair of relatively heavy dumbbells just above your knees and begin with your heels below the level of the platform so you feel a stretch in your calves. Extend your ankles to push the dumbbells up as high as you can. Squeeze your calves, then lower back down.

Shoulders/ Traps→

MILITARY PRESS ↓

Stand holding a barbell with an overhand grip just outside shoulder width. Begin with the bar just over your upper pecs and below your chin with a slight bend in your knees. Keeping your lower body stationary, press the bar straight overhead without locking out your elbows at the top. Slowly lower the bar back to the start position.

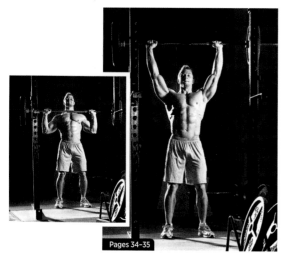

Pages 34–35

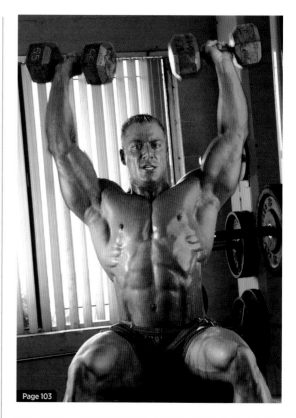

Page 103

SEATED DUMBBELL OVERHEAD PRESS

Sit on an upright bench or low-back seat and hold a set of dumbbells at shoulder level, elbows and wrists stacked. Press the weights simultaneously up and overhead until the dumbbells nearly touch, then reverse the motion to return to the start.

ARNOLD PRESS

Sit on a low-back seat holding a pair of dumbbells. Bend your elbows and hold the dumbbells at chin level with your palms and forearms facing you, not forward. Press the dumbbells overhead while simultaneously rotating your forearms until they face forward at the top of the movement. Slowly lower the weights back to the start position.

SEATED BARBELL OVERHEAD PRESS

Sit on an upright bench or low-back seat with a barbell racked overhead. Grasp the bar just outside shoulder width, lift it off the rack (preferably with the help of a spotter) and begin with it overhead, arms extended. Slowly lower the bar in front of your face until it reaches about chin level, then explosively press it back up without locking out your elbows.

UPRIGHT ROW ↓

Stand holding a barbell in front of you with a shoulder-width grip and your arms extended. Lift the bar straight up along your body by bending your elbows and contracting your delts until it reaches chest level. Hold the contraction for a count, then slowly lower the bar to full-elbow extension. Upright rows can also be performed with dumbbells using the same technique.

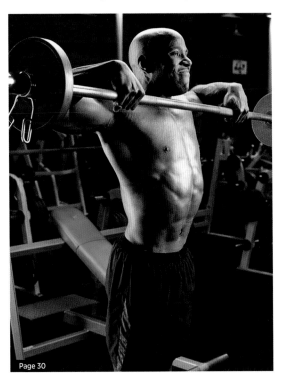

Page 30

SMITH MACHINE UPRIGHT ROW

Stand in a Smith machine holding the bar in front of your thighs with a shoulder-width grip, arms extended. Lift the bar straight up along your body by bending your elbows and contracting your delts until it reaches upper-chest level. Hold the contraction, then slowly lower the bar to full extension.

DUMBBELL LATERAL RAISE →

Stand holding a pair of relatively light dumbbells, arms at your sides. Lift the weights out in an arc until your arms are parallel to the floor. Hold the contraction for a count, then slowly lower the dumbbells back to your sides.

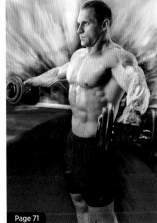

Page 71

MACHINE OVERHEAD PRESS

Adjust the seat so your upper arms are just past parallel to the floor and grasp the handles slightly outside shoulder width. Press the weight up just shy of locking out your elbows, then slowly return the weight to the start position without letting the weight rest on the stack between reps.

BENT-OVER LATERAL RAISE

Hold a pair of dumbbells and lean forward at the waist so your torso is nearly parallel to the floor. Let your arms hang straight down, elbows extended and palms facing in; keep your chest up and back flat to avoid injury. Simultaneously lift the dumbbells in an arc out to your sides until your arms are roughly parallel to the floor. (Keep your elbows relatively straight; bending them excessively takes tension off your rear delts.) Lower the weights under control to the start position; don't let them just drop.

SHOULDERS/TRAPS →

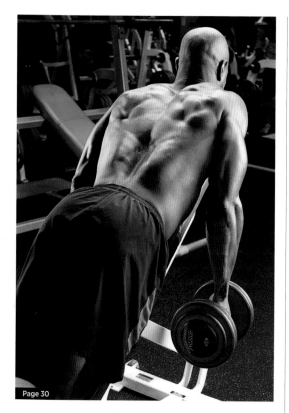

Page 30

DUMBBELL SHRUG

Stand erect with soft knees and hold a set of dumbbells outside your thighs. Slowly contract through your traps to pull your shoulders toward your ears. Hold for a second at the top, then return to the start.

MACHINE LATERAL RAISE

Sit on the seat of a lateral-raise machine so that your shoulders line up with the machine's axes of rotation. Depending on the type of machine, either grasp the handles or place your elbows on the pads with your upper arms pointed toward the floor. Contract your delts to lift your arms in an arc out to your sides until your upper arms are parallel to the floor. Pause, then slowly lower to the start position.

DUMBBELL FRONT RAISE

Hold two dumbbells in front of your thighs with your arms extended. The movement can be performed using both arms simultaneously or one at a time. If you do one-arm reps, raise one dumbbell outward in front of you, keeping your elbow extended but not locked out, until your arm is about parallel to the floor. Lower the weight back to the start position under control, then do a rep with the opposite arm. Alternate arms until you complete the desired number of reps.

REVERSE PEC-DECK FLYE

Sit backward at a pec-deck machine and grasp the handles in front of you with a neutral grip (palms facing each other). Keep your abs tight and your chest up. Flex your rear delts, keeping a slight bend in your elbows, to pull the handles back until your upper arms are just past perpendicular to your torso. Hold briefly, then return to the start position.

BARBELL SHRUG

Hold a barbell at arm's length in front of your thighs. Keeping your elbows extended, simply elevate your shoulders as high as you can — straight up and down, not backward or forward — and squeeze at the top. Lower back to the start position, depressing your shoulders, then repeat for reps.

← DUMBBELL INCLINE SHRUG

Set an incline bench to a 35–40-degree angle. Kneel on the seat with your chest flush against the bench back. Hold a dumbbell in each hand with a neutral (palms facing in) grip, arms hanging straight down. Shrug your shoulders as high as possible, squeeze your traps for a count or two, then slowly lower the dumbbells straight down to the start position.

SMITH MACHINE SHRUG

Stand directly behind the bar with your feet about shoulder-width apart. Grasp the bar with an overhand grip, hands just outside your hips. Rotate the bar to unrack it. Keeping your arms straight, chest up and eyes focused forward, raise your shoulders toward your ears. Hold the peak contraction and squeeze for a count before lowering the bar to the start position. Repeat for reps.

Triceps →

CABLE KICKBACK

Grasp the rubber ball on the low-pulley cable and align your working-side shoulder with the weight stack. Bend over until your torso is almost parallel to the floor, raise your upper arm so it's level with your torso and keep it pressed against your side. Holding your upper arm in place, extend your elbow to move your forearm up and back. Squeeze the triceps at full-arm extension, then slowly lower to the start position. Repeat for reps, then switch arms.

MACHINE DIP

Sit on the seat of the machine so your back is flat against the backpad. Grasp the handles (palms down) and begin with your elbows bent more than 90 degrees and in tight at your sides. Contract your triceps to extend your arms and press your hands down toward the floor. Squeeze your triceps hard at full extension, then slowly lower back to the start position.

TATE PRESS

Lie faceup on a flat bench holding a pair of relatively light dumbbells with your arms extended toward the ceiling, palms facing forward and the ends of the dumbbells touching over your chest. Keeping your elbows pointed out to the sides and the ends of the dumbbells touching, bend your elbows to lower the dumbbells to your chest, your palms still facing

forward. Contract your triceps to extend your arms to the start position.

CLOSE-GRIP BENCH PRESS

Position yourself as you would when benching, but grasp the bar (loaded with a lighter weight than you'd use for a normal bench) with your hands 6–12 inches apart. Lower the bar to your mid-to-lower chest, then press it back up explosively, keeping your elbows as close to your sides as possible. You can also perform this exercise using a Smith machine.

PUSHDOWN ↓

Stand facing a cable station and attach a straight bar, EZ-bar, V-bar or rope handle to a high-pulley cable. Grasp

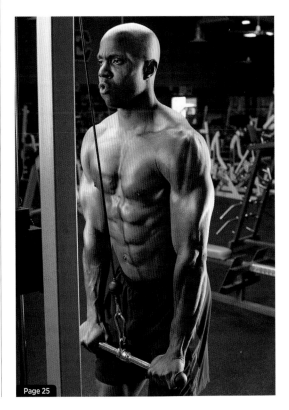

Page 25

TRICEPS →

the attachment with both hands, and keep your elbows tight at your sides and your forearms just shy of parallel to the floor. Extend your arms until they're straight, squeezing your triceps at the bottom of the rep.

REVERSE-GRIP BENCH PRESS

Lie faceup on a flat bench with a rack and grasp a barbell with a shoulder-width, reverse grip. Begin holding the bar directly above your chest with your arms extended. Keeping your elbows in, slowly lower the bar to your lower pecs. When it touches your chest, press the bar straight up to full-arm extension.

DUMBBELL LYING TRICEPS EXTENSION

Lie faceup on a flat bench and hold a pair of dumbbell at arm's length straight above you. Keeping your elbows

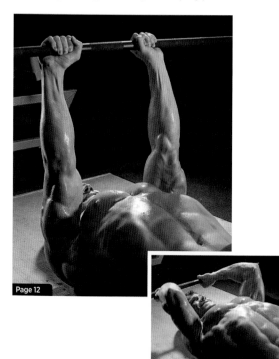

Page 12

pulled together, lower the dumbbells slowly toward your forehead. When your elbows are slightly past 90 degrees, immediately press the weights back up to the start position by contracting your triceps.

↙ "DEAD-STOP" LYING TRICEPS EXTENSION

Lie faceup on a flat bench, holding a weighted EZ-bar at arm's length over your face. Keeping your elbows pulled in, slowly lower the bar toward the top of your head. Before it touches, pause, then contract your triceps to press the weight back up to the start position. You can also perform this exercise on an incline bench.

CABLE → OVERHEAD TRICEPS EXTENSION

Attach a rope to a high-pulley cable. Sit facing away from the stack, grasp the rope near the knots and hold the attachment behind your head. Lean forward at the waist slightly. Bend your elbows less than 90 degrees. Keeping your elbows pressed

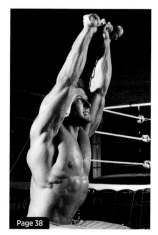

Page 38

together, extend your arms so your hands move forward and up. Squeeze your triceps hard at full-arm extension by turning your palms out at the top, then return to the start.

SEATED DUMBBELL OVERHEAD TRICEPS EXTENSION

Sit on a low-back seat with your feet flat on the floor. Grasp the inner plate of a dumbbell with both hands and hold it overhead with your elbows extended. Bending only your elbows, lower the weight behind your head until your arms form 90-degree angles. Press back up to full-arm extension and squeeze your triceps hard at the top.

Muscle-building Foods

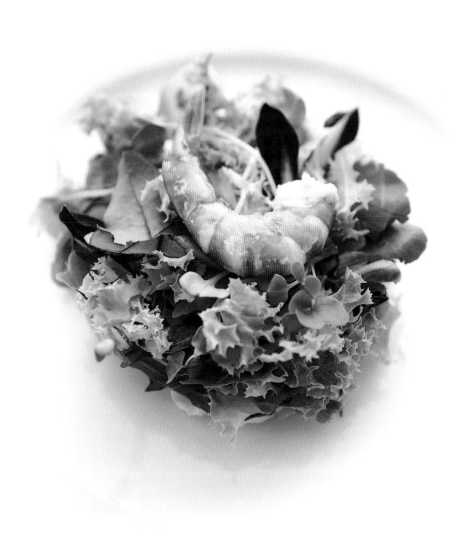

No amount of squats, bench presses, rows or curls will net you any appreciable growth in the absence of quality fuel. Use this list of 200 muscle-friendly foods to provide the foundation of your nutrition regimen, to discover new sources of protein and carbohydrates, and, most important, to track your daily macro-nutrient and calorie intake. Recording what you eat may be a pain, but it's the surest way to ensure your diet is on track. If you're indeed serious about building muscle, you won't want to leave anything to chance.

Meat→

	CALORIES	PROTEIN (G)	CARBS (G)	FAT (G)
Beef (raw unless otherwise noted)				
8 oz. beefalo (composite of cuts)	328	56	0	11
8 oz. beef brisket	352	48	0	17
8 oz. corned beef	448	32	0	34
8 oz. flank steak	352	48	0	16
4 oz. ground beef, 95% lean	152	24	0	6
4 oz. ground beef, 90% lean	196	24	0	11
4 oz. ground beef, 85% lean	240	20	0	17
4 oz. ground beef, 80% lean	284	20	0	22
4 oz. ground beef, 75% lean	328	16	0	28
4 oz. ground beef, 70% lean	372	16	0	34
1 oz. beef jerky	116	9	3	7
8 oz. beef liver	312	48	0	8
8 oz. porterhouse steak	560	43	0	42
3 large beef ribs	474	34	0	37
4 oz. roast beef	106	14	1	5
8 oz. top sirloin	456	48	0	29
8 oz. T-bone steak	496	44	0	35
8 oz. tenderloin	560	48	0	25
8 oz. tri-tip	372	47	0	19
Lamb (raw unless otherwise noted)				
4 oz. ground lamb	320	20	0	27
8 oz. lamb chops	472	40	0	32
8 oz. leg of lamb	472	40	0	32
Pork (raw unless otherwise noted)				
3 slices bacon	311	8	0	31
1 large pork chop	205	20	0	13
4 oz. ground pork	300	20	0	24
8 oz. cured ham	464	48	0	30
4 oz. smoked deli ham	186	21	1	11
1 rack baby-back ribs (roasted)	810	53	0	65
1 Italian sausage	391	16	1	35
1 smoked sausage link	265	15	1	22
8 oz. pork tenderloin	312	48	0	12

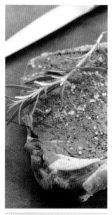
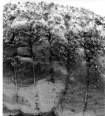
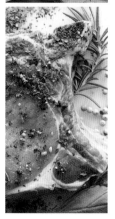

Poultry→

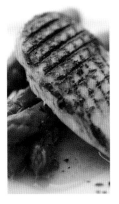

	CALORIES	PROTEIN (G)	CARBS (G)	FAT (G)
Poultry (raw unless otherwise noted)				
6 oz. chicken breast	185	39	0	2
4 oz. deli chicken breast	95	21	0	1
1 chicken thigh	82	14	0	3
6 chicken wings (Buffalo wings)	366	34	6	22
1 cornish game hen (roasted)	295	51	0	9
6 oz. duck, domesticated (meat only)	226	31	0	10
4 oz. ground ostrich	188	23	0	10
6 oz. turkey breast	189	42	0	1
4 oz. deli turkey	104	22	2	0
4 oz. ground turkey	170	20	0	9
1 oz. turkey jerky	101	19	1	1
Eggs (raw unless otherwise noted)				
1 whole large	74	6	0	5
1 whole extra large	85	7	0	6
1 whole jumbo	96	8	0	6
1 large egg white	17	4	0	0

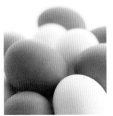

Dairy→

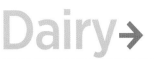

	CALORIES	PROTEIN (G)	CARBS (G)	FAT (G)
Cheese				
1 slice low-fat American	38	5	1	1
1 slice cheddar	113	7	0	9
8 oz. low-fat cottage cheese (1%)	163	28	6	2
8 oz. cottage cheese (small curd)	232	28	6	10
1 slice low-fat Monterey jack	88	8	0	6
1 oz. mozzarella, part skim	72	7	1	5
1 slice provolone	98	7	1	7
1 slice low-fat Swiss	50	8	1	1
Milk				
8 oz. fat-free	83	8	12	0
8 oz. low-fat (1%)	102	8	12	2
8 oz. reduced-fat (2%)	122	8	11	5
8 oz. whole (3.25%)	146	8	11	8
1 Tbsp. fat-free sour cream	11	0	2	0
1 Tbsp. reduced-fat sour cream	20	0	1	2
Yogurt				
8 oz. fat-free (fruit)	213	10	43	0
8 oz. low-fat (fruit)	225	9	42	3
8 oz. low-fat (plain)	143	12	16	4

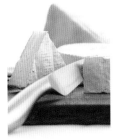
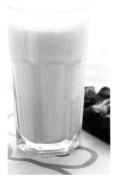

Muscle-building Foods

Seafood→

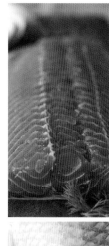

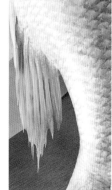

	CALORIES	PROTEIN (G)	CARBS (G)	FAT (G)
Seafood (raw unless otherwise noted)				
6 oz. bass	194	32	0	6
6 oz. catfish	230	26	0	13
6 medium clams	66	11	2	1
6 oz. cod	140	30	0	1
1 crab cake	160	11	5	10
1 Alaskan king crab leg	144	31	0	1
1 Dungeness crab	140	28	1	2
3 oz. eel (mixed species)	156	16	0	10
6 oz. flounder	154	32	0	2
6 oz. haddock	148	32	0	1
6 oz. halibut	188	36	0	4
1 medium lobster	135	28	1	1
6 oz. mackerel (mixed species)	268	34	0	13
6 medium mussels	84	11	4	2
6 medium oysters	57	6	3	2
6 oz. Atlantic salmon	312	34	0	18
1 can sardines (in oil, drained)	191	23	0	11
6 oz. scallops	150	28	0	2
6 oz. sea bass	164	32	0	3
6 oz. sole	154	32	0	2
4 oz. shrimp	120	23	1	2
3 oz. fried squid (calamari)	149	15	7	6
6 oz. swordfish	206	34	0	7
6 oz. trout	252	36	0	11
1 can white tuna (in water)	220	41	0	5
1 can light tuna (in water)	191	42	0	1
6 oz. whitefish	228	32	0	10

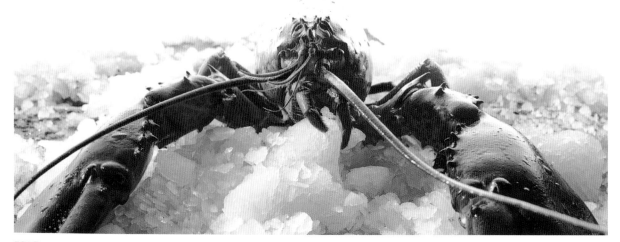

Fruits & Juices→

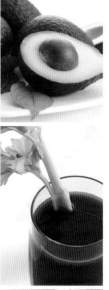

Fruits	CALORIES	PROTEIN (G)	CARBS (G)	FAT (G)
1 large apple	110	0	30	0
1 avocado	289	3	15	27
1 medium banana	105	1	27	0
1 cup blueberries	83	1	21	0
1 medium cantaloupe	188	5	45	1
1/2 large grapefruit	53	1	13	0
1 medium nectarine	60	1	14	0
1 large orange	86	2	22	0
1 medium peach	38	1	9	0
1 medium pear	96	1	26	0
1 cup sliced pineapple	79	1	20	0
1 cup raspberries	64	1	15	1
1 cup strawberries, whole	46	1	11	0
Juices				
8 oz. apple juice (unsweetened)	117	0	29	0
8 oz. grapefruit juice	96	1	23	0
8 oz. orange juice	110	2	25	1
8 oz. tomato juice	41	2	10	0

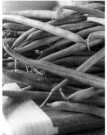

Vegetables→

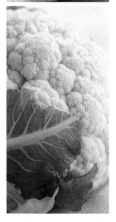

Vegetables	CALORIES	PROTEIN (G)	CARBS (G)	FAT (G)
20 asparagus spears	60	6	12	0
1 can green beans	52	3	12	0
1 cup chopped broccoli	31	3	6	0
1 cup Brussels sprouts	38	3	8	0
1 medium carrot	25	1	6	0
1 cup chopped cauliflower	28	1	3	0
1 medium celery stalk	6	0	1	0
1 cup canned corn	133	4	30	2
1 cup chopped eggplant	20	1	5	0
1 medium onion	46	1	11	0
1 cup peas	118	8	21	1
1 medium baked potato	161	4	37	0
2 cups green salad	44	3	8	0
1 medium sweet potato	103	2	24	0
1 medium tomato	22	1	5	0
1/2 cup tomato sauce (marinara)	92	2	14	3
1 cup sliced zucchini, boiled	29	1	7	0

Muscle-building Foods

Grains→

	CALORIES	PROTEIN (G)	CARBS (G)	FAT (G)
Bread/Crackers				
1 medium plain bagel	289	11	56	2
1 medium bran muffin	305	8	55	8
1 plain dinner roll	84	2	14	2
1 plain English muffin	134	4	26	1
1 whole-wheat English muffin	134	6	27	1
1 plain hamburger roll	120	4	21	2
1 slice multigrain bread	65	3	12	1
1 large pita pocket (white, 6.5")	165	5	33	1
1 large pita pocket (wheat, 6.5")	170	6	35	2
1 slice pumpernickel bread	65	2	12	1
1 slice rye bread	83	3	15	1
6 saltine crackers	154	3	26	4
1 slice white bread	66	2	13	1
1 slice whole-wheat bread	70	3	13	1
6 whole-wheat crackers	108	2	18	4
Cereal				
1 cup Cheerios	111	4	22	2
1 cup Corn Flakes	101	2	24	0
1 cup corn grits, cooked	143	3	31	0
1 packet Cream of Wheat (instant)	102	3	22	0
1/2 cup Grape-Nuts	208	6	47	1
1 cup cooked oatmeal	147	6	25	2
1 cup Raisin Bran	178	5	43	1
1 cup Rice Krispies	108	2	24	0
1 cup Special K	117	7	22	0
1 cup Wheaties	106	3	24	1
Pasta (cooked)				
1 cup couscous	176	6	36	0
1 cup egg noodles	221	7	40	3
1 cup macaroni and cheese	370	16	68	4
1 cup rice noodles	192	2	44	0
1 cup soba	113	6	24	0
1 cup spaghetti	221	8	43	1
1 cup whole-wheat pasta	174	7	37	1
Rice (cooked)				
1 cup brown (medium grain)	218	5	46	2
1 rice cake	35	1	7	0
1 cup white (medium grain)	242	4	53	0
1 cup white (long grain)	205	4	45	0
1 cup wild	166	7	35	1

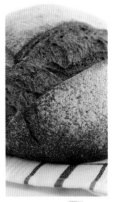

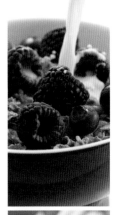

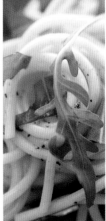

Legumes & Nuts →

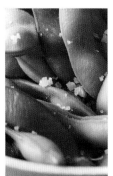

	CALORIES	PROTEIN (G)	CARBS (G)	FAT (G)
Legumes (cooked)				
1 cup baked beans	239	12	54	1
1 cup black beans	227	15	41	1
1 cup chickpeas	286	12	54	3
1 cup edamame (soybeans)	254	22	20	12
½ cup hummus	207	10	18	12
1 cup kidney beans	225	15	40	1
1 cup lima beans	216	15	39	1
1 cup navy beans	255	15	47	1
1 Tbsp. peanut butter	94	4	3	8
1 oz. peanuts	166	7	6	14
1 cup pinto beans	245	15	45	1
1 cup refried beans	237	14	39	3
Nuts				
1 oz. almonds	169	6	5	15
1 oz. cashews	163	4	9	13
1 oz. hazelnuts	183	4	5	18
1 oz. macadamia nuts	203	2	4	22
1 oz. mixed nuts	168	5	7	15
1 oz. pecans	201	3	4	21
1 oz. English walnuts	185	4	4	18

Miscellaneous →

	CALORIES	PROTEIN (G)	CARBS (G)	FAT (G)
Condiments				
1 Tbsp. jams and preserves	56	0	14	0
1 Tbsp. ketchup	15	0	4	0
1 Tbsp. fat-free mayo	11	0	2	0
1 Tbsp. light mayo	50	0	1	5
1 Tbsp. regular mayo	57	0	4	5
1 tsp. or packet mustard	3	0	0	0
1 Tbsp. fat-free Italian dressing	10	0	2	0
1 Tbsp. olive oil	119	0	0	14
1 Tbsp. oil/vinegar dressing	72	0	0	8
1 tsp. sugar	16	0	4	0
Soups/Stews/Chili (cooked unless otherwise noted)				
1 cup beef broth	29	5	2	0
1 cup beef stew	222	111	6	13
1 cup black bean	116	62	0	2
1 cup chicken broth	5	1	0	0
1 cup chicken noodle	76	6	9	2
1 cup chili with beans	287	15	30	14
1 cup minestrone	82	4	11	3
1 cup New England clam chowder	117	5	20	2
1 package dry Ramen noodles	385	8	56	15
1 cup split pea with ham	190	10	28	4
1 cup tomato	85	2	17	2

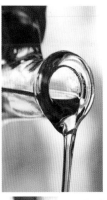

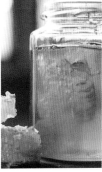